*Gary Holden, DSW*
*Gary Rosenberg, PhD*
*Kathleen Barker, PhD*
*Editors*

# Bibliometrics in Social Work

*Bibliometrics in Social Work* has been co-published simultaneously as *Social Work in Health Care,* Volume 41, Numbers 3/4 2005.

*Pre-publication*
*REVIEWS,*
*COMMENTARIES,*
*EVALUATIONS . . .*

"A THOUGHT-PROVOKING CALL TO ACTION. . . . The editors provide us with a careful review of the pros and cons of bibliometrics and warn us of the drawbacks of over-reliance on these methods. The opening chapters and the rebuttal are excellent sources for the state of knowledge production in social work. . . . The third chapter is also a must-read for any social work dean or director, as well as any relevant promotion and tenure committees."

**Ram A. Cnaan, PhD**
*Professor and Associate Dean*
*for Research and Doctoral Education*
*and Director*
*Program for Religion and Social Policy*
*Research*
*School of Social Policy and Practice*
*University of Pennsylvania*

*More Pre-publication
REVIEWS, COMMENTARIES, EVALUATIONS . . .*

"This is THE MOST COHERENT AND TECHNICALLY ACCURATE WORK that I have seen to date that enunciates and clarifies both the potential and the limitations of the state of bibliometrics affairs in social work. Few efforts until now have demonstrated this kind of intellectual integrity; it is indeed refreshing. The authors advance our understanding and use of citation analysis in the evaluation of scholarship and scholars in social work. The book includes excellent critiques by some of the major thinkers in the field who raise important and, at times, thorny questions.

Subsequently, the authors competently and respectfully address the issues raised. THIS FORMAT, DONE THIS WELL, SHOULD BECOME THE STANDARD VEHICLE FOR ADVANCING THE SCIENCE OF SOCIAL work if we are to gain equal footing with other social science disciplines in contributing to the wider knowledge base."

**William S. Rowe, DSW**
*Professor and Director
School of Social Work
University of South Florida*

The Haworth Social Work Practice Press
An Imprint of The Haworth Press, Inc.

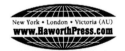

# Bibliometrics in Social Work

*Bibliometrics in Social Work* has been co-published simultaneously as *Social Work in Health Care*, Volume 41, Numbers 3/4 2005.

ALL HAWORTH SOCIAL WORK PRACTICE PRESS
BOOKS AND JOURNALS ARE PRINTED ON
CERTIFIED ACID-FREE PAPER

# Bibliometrics in Social Work

Gary Holden, DSW
Gary Rosenberg, PhD
Kathleen Barker, PhD
Editors

Gary Rosenberg, PhD
Andrew Weissman, PhD
Series Editors

*Bibliometrics in Social Work* has been co-published simultaneously as *Social Work in Health Care*, Volume 41, Numbers 3/4 2005.

The Haworth Social Work Practice Press
An Imprint of The Haworth Press, Inc.

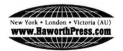

Published by

The Haworth Social Work Practice Press, 10 Alice Street, Binghamton, NY 13904-1580 USA

The Haworth Social Work Practice Press is an imprint of The Haworth Press, Inc., 10 Alice Street, Binghamton, NY 13904-1580 USA.

*Bibliometrics in Social Work* has been co-published simultaneously as *Social Work in Health Care,* Volume 41, Numbers 3/4 2005.

© 2005 by The Haworth Press, Inc. All rights reserved. No part of this work may be reproduced or utilized in any form or by any means, electronic or mechanical, including photocopying, microfilm and recording, or by any information storage and retrieval system, without permission in writing from the publisher. Printed in the United States of America.

The development, preparation, and publication of this work has been undertaken with great care. However, the publisher, employees, editors, and agents of The Haworth Press and all imprints of The Haworth Press, Inc., including The Haworth Medical Press® and The Pharmaceutical Products Press®, are not responsible for any errors contained herein or for consequences that may ensue from use of materials or information contained in this work. Opinions expressed by the author(s) are not necessarily those of The Haworth Press, Inc.

Cover design by Marylouise E. Doyle

**Library of Congress Cataloging-in-Publication Data**

Bibliometrics in Social Work/ Gary Holden, DSW, Gary Rosenberg, PhD, Kathleen Barker, PhD, editors.
      p. cm.
     "Bibliometrics in Social Work has been co-published simultaneously as Social work in health care, volume 41, numbers 3/4 2005"
     Includes bibliographical references and index.
     ISBN 13: 978-0-7890-3070-2 (hard cover : alk. paper)
     ISBN 10: 0-7890-3070-5 (hard cover : alk. paper)
     ISBN 13: 978-0-7890-3071-9 (soft cover : alk paper)
     ISBN 10: 0-7890-3071-3 (soft cover : alk. paper)
     1. Social service–Statistical methods. 2. Bibliometrics. I. Holden, Gary, 1951–. II. Rosenberg, Gary. III. Barker, Kathleen, 1951– IV. Social work in health care.
HV29.B54 2005
361.3'072'7–dc22                                    2005015514

# Monographic Separates from *Social Work in Health Care*

For additional information on these and other Haworth Press titles, including descriptions, tables of contents, reviews, and prices, use the QuickSearch catalog at http://www.HaworthPress.com.

**Bibliometrics in Social Work,** edited by Gary Holden, DSW, Gary Rosenberg, PhD, and Kathleen Barker, PhD (Vol. 41, No. 3/4, 2005). *An overview of the pros and cons of using bibliometrics in social work research.*

**Social Work Visions from Around the Globe: Citizens, Methods, and Approaches,** edited by Anna Metteri, MSoc et al. (Vol. 39, No. 1/2 and 3/4, 2004) *"VALUABLE to practitioners in health and mental health . . . . Shows in a practical way how citizenship can be an inclusive practice related to social justice rather than a way of excluding people from opportunities and resources in our societies." (Heather D' Cruz, PhD, MSW, Senior Lecturer in Social Work,, School of Health and Social Development, Faculty of Health and Behavioral Sciences, Deakin University, Geelong, Victoria, Australia)*

**Social Work Health and Mental Health: Practice, Research and Programs,** edited by Alun C. Jackson, PhD, and Steven P. Segal, PhD (Vol. 34, No. 1/2 and 3/4, 2001, and Vol. 35, No. 1/2, 2002). *Explores international perspectives on social work practice in health and mental health.*

**Clinical Data-Mining in Practice-Based Research: Social Work in Hospital Settings,** edited by Irwin Epstein, PhD, and Susan Blumenfield, DSW, (Vol. 33, No. 3/4, 2001). *"Challenging and illuminating. . . . This remarkable collection of exemplary studies provides inspiration and support to social workers. This book will be valuable not only as a guide to practitioners, but also is an important addition to the teaching materials for courses in social work in health care and in social research methodology." (Kay V. Davidson, DSW, Dean and Professor, University of Connecticut School of Social Work, West Hartford)*

**Behavioral and Social Sciences in 21st Century Health Care: Contributions and Opportunities,** edited by Gary Rosenberg, PhD, and Andrew Weissman, PhD (Vol. 33, No. 1, 2001). *"Stimulating and provocative. . . . The range of topics covered makes this book an ideal reader for health care practice courses with a combined health/mental health focus." (Goldie Kadushin, PhD, Associate Professor, School of Social Welfare, University of Wisconsin-Milwaukee)*

**Seventh Doris Siegel Memorial Colloquium: Behavioral Health Care Practice in the 21st Century,** edited by Gary Rosenberg, PhD, and Andrew Weissman, PhD (Vol. 31, No. 2, 2000). *"A valuable group of research studies examining important and pertinent issues. . . . Offers a fresh perspective on critical problems encountered by health care institutions, providers, patients, and families. Excellent." (Mildred D. Mailick, DSW, Professor Emerita, Hunter College School of Social Work, City University of New York)*

**Social Work in Mental Health: Trends and Issues,** edited by Uri Aviram (Vol. 25, No. 3, 1997). *"Suggests ways to maintain social work values in a time that emphasizes cost containment and legal requirements that may result in practices and policies that are antithetical to the profession." (Phyllis Solomon, PhD, Professor, School of Social Work, University of Pennsylvania)*

**International Perspectives on Social Work in Health Care: Past, Present and Future,** edited by Gail K. Auslander, DSW (Vol. 25, No. 1/2, 1997). *"The authors explore the need for new theoretical and practice models, in addition to developments in health and social work research and administration." (Council on Social Work and Education)*

**Fundamentals of Perinatal Social Work: A Guide for Clinical Practice with Women, Infants, and Families,** edited by Regina Furlong Lind, MSW, LCSW, and Debra Honig Bachman, MSW, LCSW (Vol. 24, No. 3/4, 1997). *"A knowledge summation of the essence of perinatal social work that is long overdue. It is a must for any beginning perinatal social worker to own one!" (Charlotte Collins Bursi, MSSW, Perinatal Social Worker, University of Tennessee Newborn Center; Founding President, National Association of Perinatal Social Workers)*

***Professional Social Work Education and Health Care: Challenges for the Future,*** edited by Mildred D. Mailick, DSW, and Phyllis Caroff, DSW (Vol. 24, No. 1/2, 1996). *Responds to critical concerns about the educational preparation of social workers within the rapidly changing health care environment.*

***Social Work in Pediatrics,*** edited by Ruth B. Smith, PhD, MSW, and Helen G. Clinton, MSW (Vol. 21, No. 1, 1995). *"It presents models of service delivery and clinical practice that offer responses to the challenges of today's health care system." (Journal of Social Work Education)*

***Social Work Leadership in Healthcare: Directors' Perspectives,*** edited by Gary Rosenberg, PhD, and Andrew Weissman, DSW (Vol. 20, No. 4, 1995). *Social work managers describe their work and work environment, detailing what qualities and traits are needed to be effective and successful now and in the future.*

***Social Work in Ambulatory Care: New Implications for Health and Social Services,*** edited by Gary Rosenberg, PhD, and Andrew Weissman, DSW (Vol. 20, No. 1, 1994). *"A most timely book dealing with issues related to the current shift in health care delivery to ambulatory care and social work's need to position itself in this health care arena." (Barbara Berkman, DSW, Director of Research and Quality Assessment, Massachusetts General Hospital; Associate Director, Harvard Upper New England Geriatric Education Center, Harvard Medical School)*

***Women's Health and Social Work: Feminist Perspectives,*** edited by Miriam Meltzer Olson, DSW (Vol. 19, No. 3/4, 1994). *"[Chapters] explore how social workers can better understand and address women's health, including such conditions as breast cancer, menopause, and depression. They also discuss health care centers and African-American women and AIDS." (Reference & Research Book News)*

***The Changing Context of Social Health Care: Its Implications for Providers and Consumers,*** edited by Helen Rehr, DSW, and Gary Rosenberg, PhD (Vol. 15, No. 4, 1991). *"Required reading for every student and practitioner with a vision of improving our health care delivery system." (Candyce S. Berger, PhD, MSW, Director of Social Work, University of Washington Medical Center; Associate Professor, School of Social Work, University of Washington)*

***Social Workers in Health Care Management: The Move to Leadership,*** edited by Gary Rosenberg, PhD, and Sylvia S. Clarke, MSc, ACSW (Vol. 12, No. 3, 1988). *"Social workers interested in hospital social work management and the potential for advancement within the health care field will find the book interesting and challenging as well as helpful." (Social Thought)*

***Social Work and Genetics: A Guide to Practice,*** edited by Sylvia Schild, DSW, and Rita Beck Black, DSW (Supp #1, 1984). *"Precisely defines the responsibilities of social work in the expanding field of medical genetics and presents a clear, comprehensive overview of basic genetic principles and issues." (Health and Social Work)*

***Advancing Social Work Practice in the Health Care Field: Emerging Issues and New Perspectives,*** edited by Gary Rosenberg, PhD, and Helen Rehr, DSW (Vol. 8, No. 3, 1983). *"Excellent articles, useful bibliographies, and additional reading lists." (Australian Social Work)*

# Indexing, Abstracting & Website/Internet Coverage

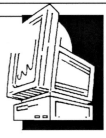

This section provides you with a list of major indexing & abstracting services and other tools for bibliographic access. That is to say, each service began covering this periodical during the year noted in the right column. Most Websites which are listed below have indicated that they will either post, disseminate, compile, archive, cite or alert their own Website users with research-based content from this work. (This list is as current as the copyright date of this publication.)

Abstracting, Website/Indexing Coverage . . . . . . . . . Year When Coverage Began

- *Abstracts in Social Gerontology: Current Literature on Aging* . . . . . . 1989
- *Academic Abstracts/CD-ROM* . . . . . . . . . . . . . . . . . . . . . . . . . . . . . . 1995
- *Academic Search Elite (EBSCO)* . . . . . . . . . . . . . . . . . . . . . . . . . . . . 2001
- *Academic Search Premier (EBSCO) <http://www.epnet.com/academic/acasearchprem.asp>* . . . . . . . . 1994
- *AgeLine Database <http://research.aarp.org/ageline>* . . . . . . . . . . . 2000
- *Applied Social Sciences Index & Abstracts (ASSIA) (Online: ASSI via Data-Star) (CDRom: ASSIA Plus) <http://www.csa.com>* . . . . . . . . . . . . . . . . . . . . . . . . . . . . . . . . . . 1987
- *Behavioral Medicine Abstracts (Annals of Behavioral Medicine)* . . . . 1983
- *Behavioral Medicine Abstracts (Pain Evaluation and Treatment Institute)* . . . . . . . . . . . . . . . . . . . . . . . . . . . . . . . . . . . . . . . . . . . 1997
- *Business Source Corporate: coverage of nearly 3,350 quality magazines and journals; designed to meet the diverse information needs of corporation; EBSCO Publishing <http://www.epnet.com/corporate/bsourcecorp.asp>* . . 1994
- *CareData: the database supporting social care management and pratice <http://www.elsc.org.uk/caredata/caredata.htm>* . . . . 1975
- *CINAHL (Cumulative Index to Nursing & Allied Health Literature), in print, EBSCO, and SilverPlatter, Data-Star, and PaperChase. (Support materials include Subject Heading List, Database Search Guide, and instructional video) <http://www.cinahl.com>* . . . . . . . . . . . . . . . . . . . . . . . . . . . . . . 1981

(continued)

- *Current Contents/Social & Behavioral Sciences* <http://www.isinet.com>..................................... 1999
- *e-psyche, LLC* <http://www.e-psyche.net> ...................... 2001
- *EBSCOHost Electronic Journals Service (EJS)* <http://ejournals.ebsco.com>............................. 2001
- *Educational Research Abstracts (ERA) (online database)* <http://www.tandf.co.uk/era>............................. 1991
- *EMBASE.com (The Power of EMBASE + MEDLINE Combined)* <http://www.embase.com> ............................... 1975
- *EMBASE/Excerpta Medica Secondary Publishing Division. Included in newsletters, review journals, major reference works, magazines & abstract journals* <http://www.elsevier.nl>........ 1975
- *Excerpta Medica ... See EMBASE* ........................... 1975
- *Family & Society Studies Worldwide* <http://www.nisc.com> ...... 2001
- *Family Index Database* <http://www.familyscholar.com> ......... 1995
- *Family Violence & Sexual Assault Bulletin*..................... 1999
- *Google* <http://www.google.com>............................. 2004
- *Google Scholar* <http://scholar.google.com> ................... 2004
- *Haworth Document Delivery Center* <http://www.HaworthPress.com/journals/dds.asp> .......... 2004
- *Health & Psychological Instruments (HaPI) Database (available through online and as a CD-ROM from Ovid Technologies)*................................. 1986
- *Health Source: Indexing & Abstracting of 160 selected health related journals, updated monthly: EBSCO Publishing* ... 1995
- *Health Source Plus: expanded version of "Health Source": EBSCO Publishing* ...................................... 1995
- *Human Resources Abstracts (HRA)* ......................... 1992
- *IBZ International Bibliography of Periodical Literature* <http://www.saur.de>................................... 1995
- *Index Guide to College Journals (core list compiled by integrating 48 indexes frequently used to support undergraduate programs in small to medium sized libraries)* ...................... 1999
- *Index Medicus (National Library of Medicine) ... (print edition ceased ... see instead MEDLINE)* <http://www.nlm.nih.gov>............................... 1992
- *Index to Periodical Articles Related to Law* <http://www.law.utexas.edu>............................. 1991
- *Internationale Bibliographie der geistes- und sozialwissenschaftlichen Zeitschriftenliteratur... See IBZ* <http:www.saur.de> ................................... 1995
- *ISI Web of Science* <http://www.isinet.com> ................... 2003
- *Journal of Social Work Practice "Abstracts Section"* <http:www.carfax.co.uk/jsw-ad.htm> ..................... 2000

(continued)

- *Links@Ovid (via CrossRef targeted DOI links) <http://www.ovid.com>* .................................. 2005
- *Magazines for Libraries (Katz)... (see 2003 edition)* ............. 2003
- *MasterFILE Elite: coverage of nearly 1,200 periodicals covering general reference, business, health, education, general science, multi-cultural issues and much more; EBSCO Publishing <http://www.epnet.com/government/mfelite.asp>* ............... 1994
- *MasterFILE Premier: coverage of more than 1,950 periodicals covering general reference, business, health, education, general science, multi-cultural issues and much more; EBSCO Publishing <http://www.epnet.com/government/mfpremier.asp>* ........ 1994
- *MasterFILE Select: coverage of nearly 770 periodicals covering general reference, business, health, education, general science, multi-cultural issues and much more; EBSCO Publishing <http://www.epnet.com/government/mfselect.asp>* ............ 2003
- *MEDLINE (National Library of Medicine) <http://www.nlm.nih.gov>* ............................... 2001
- *OCLC ArticleFirst <http://www.oclc.org/services/databases/>* ..... 2002
- *OVID HealthSTAR* ........................................ 1997
- *Ovid Linksolver (OpenURL link resolver via CrossRef targeted DOI links) <http://www.linksolver.com>* ..... 2005
- *ProQuest Research Library. Contents of this publication are indexed and abstracted in the ProQuest Research Library database (includes only abstracts ... not full-text), available on ProQuest Information & Learning <http://www.proquest.com>* ........ 2004
- *Psychological Abstracts (PsycINFO) <http.www.apa.org>* ........ 1975
- *PubMed <http://www.ncbi.nlm.nih.gov/pubmed/>* ............... 2000
- *Referativnyi Zhurnal (Abstracts Journal of the All-Russian Institute of Scientific and Technical Information–in Russian) <http://www.viniti.ru* ................................... 1992
- *RESEARCH ALERT/ISI Alerting Services <http://www.isinet.com>* ................................ 2000
- *Sexual Diversity Studies: Gay, Lesbian, Bisexual & Transgender Abstracts (formerly Gay & Lesbian Abstracts) provides comprehensive & in-depth coverage of the world's GLBT literature compiled by NISC & published on the Internet & CD-ROM <http://www.nisc.com>* ..... 1977
- *Social Sciences Citation Index (ISI) <http://www.isinet.com>* ...... 2000
- *Social Scisearch <http://www.isinet.com>* .................... 2000
- *Social Services Abstracts <http://www.csa.com>* ................ 1990

(continued)

- *Social Work Abstracts <http://www.silverplatter.com/catalog/swab.htm>* ................................. 1982
- *Social Work Acess Network (SWAN) <http://cosw.sc.edu/swan/media.html>* ..................... 2005
- *Sociological Abstracts (SA) <http://www.csa.com>* ............... 1990
- *Special Educational Needs Abstracts* ........................ 1989
- *Studies on Women and Gender Abstracts <http:www.tandf.co.uk/swa>* ............................. 1993
- *SwetsWise <http://www.swets.com>* .......................... 2001
- *Violence and Abuse Abstracts: A Review of Current Literature on Interpersonal Violence (VAA)* .......................... 1995
- *zetoc <http://zetoc.mimas.ac.uk/>* ............................. 2004

*Special Bibliographic Notes related to special journal issues (separates) and indexing/abstracting:*

- indexing/abstracting services in this list will also cover material in any "separate" that is co-published simultaneously with Haworth's special thematic journal issue or DocuSerial. Indexing/abstracting usually covers material at the article/chapter level.
- monographic co-editions are intended for either non-subscribers or libraries which intend to purchase a second copy for their circulating collections.
- monographic co-editions are reported to all jobbers/wholesalers/approval plans. The source journal is listed as the "series" to assist the prevention of duplicate purchasing in the same manner utilized for books-in-series.
- to facilitate user/access services all indexing/abstracting services are encouraged to utilize the co-indexing entry note indicated at the bottom of the first page of each article/chapter/contribution.
- this is intended to assist a library user of any reference tool (whether print, electronic, online, or CD-ROM) to locate the monographic version if the library has purchased this version but not a subscription to the source journal.
- individual articles/chapters in any Haworth publication are also available through the Haworth Document Delivery Service (HDDS).

# Bibliometrics in Social Work

## CONTENTS

Tracing Thought Through Time and Space: A Selective Review
of Bibliometrics in Social Work     1
*Gary Holden, DSW*
*Gary Rosenberg, PhD*
*Kathleen Barker, PhD*

What Happens to Our Ideas? A Bibliometric Analysis
of Articles in *Social Work in Health Care* in the 1990s     35
*Gary Rosenberg, PhD*
*Gary Holden, DSW*
*Kathleen Barker, PhD*

Bibliometrics: A Potential Decision Making Aid in Hiring,
Reappointment, Tenure and Promotion Decisions     67
*Gary Holden, DSW*
*Gary Rosenberg, PhD*
*Kathleen Barker, PhD*

Following in the Footnotes of Giants:
Citation Analysis and Its Discontents     93
*Irwin Epstein, PhD*

The Paradox of Faculty Publications in Professional Journals     103
*Robert G. Green, PhD*

Politics of Personnel and Landscapes of Knowledge     109
*Stuart A. Kirk, PhD*

Bibliometrics: The Best Available Information?     117
*Waldo C. Klein, PhD, MSW*
*Martin Bloom, PhD*

Bibliometrics and Social Work:
   A Two-Edged Sword Can Still Be a Blunt Instrument    123
     *Jan Ligon, PhD*
     *Bruce A. Thyer, PhD*

Shallow Science or Meta-Cognitive Insights:
   A Few Thoughts on Reflection via Bibliometrics    129
     *Gary Holden, DSW*
     *Gary Rosenberg, PhD*
     *Kathleen Barker, PhD*

Index    149

# ABOUT THE EDITORS

**Gary Holden, DSW,** is currently Professor at the New York University School of Social Work. He was formerly on the faculty of the Mount Sinai School of Medicine. He received his masters in social work in 1987 and doctorate in social welfare (with distinction) in 1990 from Columbia University. Dr. Holden is the editor of *Information for Practice*, the professional research dissemination blog for social service professionals throughout the world (http://www.nyu.edu/socialwork/ ip/). He is a member of the Editorial Boards of *Social Work in Health Care* and the *Journal of Social Work Education*. Dr. Holden has over eighty publications on a range of topics including behavioral health and telehealth, research methodology, social work education, and the Social Cognitive Theory construct self-efficacy.

**Gary Rosenberg, PhD,** is currently the Edith J. Baerwald Professor of Community and Preventive Medicine, Mount Sinai School of Medicine. Dr. Rosenberg is the recipient of numerous awards–the Outstanding Alumni Award from Hunter College and Adelphia University, and the Founders Day Award from New York University. In 2004, NASW's New York City Chapter inducted Dr. Rosenberg as an NASW Social Work Pioneer. He is a fellow of the New York Academy of Medicine and is the President of the Board of the Center for Social Administration, a post-master's management education institute, President of the Board of Senior Health Partners, and agency serving the aging population of New York and a memeber of the Board of Directors of Union Settlement and Job Path. Dr. Rosenberg is the Editor-in-Chief of two peer-reveiewed journals on health policy and practices and on mental health. He has written or edited 12 books, 22 book chapters and is the author of over 60 articles in professional journals.

**Kathleen Barker, PhD,** Professor of Psychology, is a social psychologist who conducts multi-disciplinary research in the areas of nonstandard work, higher education and social justice, as well as on methodological issues. She co-edited a collection *Contingent Work: American Employment Relations in Transition*. She recently served on the American Psychological Association's Workforce Analysis Task Force. She has published sole and co-authored chapters on workplace issues and has published articles in *Sex Roles, Psychological Reports, Social Work and Education, and Social Work in Health Care*. Dr. Baker has served in instructional and administrative capacities at Bard College, Columbia University, New York University, Pace University, and most recently Medgar Evers College of The City University of New York. She received her doctorate in Social Personality Psychology in 1990 from The Graduate Center of The City University of New York.

# Tracing Thought Through Time and Space: A Selective Review of Bibliometrics in Social Work

Gary Holden, DSW
Gary Rosenberg, PhD
Kathleen Barker, PhD

**SUMMARY.** Bibliometrics is a field of research that examines bodies of knowledge within and across disciplines. Citation analysis, a component of bibliometrics, focuses on the quantitative assessment of citation patterns within a body of literature. Citation analysis has been used in social work to examine the quantity and the impact of the work of indi-

---

Gary Holden is Professor, New York University of Social Work. Gary Rosenberg is Edith J. Baerwald Professor of Community and Preventive Medicine, Mount Sinai School of Medicine. Kathleen Barker is Professor of Psychology, The City University of New York: Medgar Evers College.

Address correspondence to: Gary Holden, DSW, Room 407, MC: 6112, New York University: School of Social Work, 1 Washington Square North, New York, NY 10003 (E-mail: gary.holden@nyu.edu).

[Haworth co-indexing entry note]: "Tracing Thought Through Time and Space: A Selective Review of Bibliometrics in Social Work." Holden, Gary, Gary Rosenberg, and Kathleen Barker. Co-published simultaneously in *Social Work in Health Care* (The Haworth Social Work Practice Press, an imprint of The Haworth Press, Inc.) Vol. 41, No. 3/4, 2005, pp. 1-34; and: *Bibliometrics in Social Work* (ed: Gary Holden, Gary Rosenberg and Kathleen Barker) The Haworth Social Work Practice Press, an imprint of The Haworth Press, Inc., 2005, pp. 1-34. Single or multiple copies of this article are available for a fee from The Haworth Document Delivery Service [1-800-HAWORTH, 9:00 a.m. - 5:00 p.m. (EST). E-mail address: docdelivery@haworthpress.com].

Available online at http://www.haworthpress.com/web/SWHC
© 2005 by The Haworth Press, Inc. All rights reserved.
doi:10.1300/J010v41n03_01

viduals and academic institutions. This paper presents a selective review of these uses of bibliometrics within social work. *[Article copies available for a fee from The Haworth Document Delivery Service: 1-800-HAWORTH. E-mail address: <docdelivery@haworthpress.com> Website: <http://www.HaworthPress.com> © 2005 by The Haworth Press, Inc. All rights reserved.]*

**KEYWORDS.** Informetrics, scientometrics, citation analysis, sociology of science, social work education

## INTRODUCTION TO BIBLIOMETRICS

Scholarship in social work has been examined from a variety of perspectives (e.g., Fraser, 1994). One of those perspectives uses bibliometrics, a field of research that examines bodies of knowledge within and across disciplines (Norton, 2000; Twining, 2002). Rao (1998) notes that a variety of terms have been used over time and across disparate geographic locales to refer to relatively similar areas of study, such as statistical bibliography, librametry, scientometrics and informetrics. More recently, the terms webometrics and cybermetrics have been observed (Nisonger, 2001). Nisonger states that the 'metrics' in these various descriptions of research areas refers to quantitative assessments of the topic (e.g., scientometrics involves the quantitative analysis of science). Informetrics is the more general field of study that encompasses scientometrics and bibliometrics (Bar-Ilan, 2001; Brookes, 1990; Tague-Sutcliffe, 1992). The term bibliometrics will be used here as it is the one to which social workers will most likely have been exposed.

Bibliometrics draw on a variety of theories and models. These include: information science and cybernetics (Brookes, 1991); the sociology of science (e.g., Robert Merton's group at Columbia: Cole, 2000); an economic theory of science (e.g., Franck, 2002); semiotics (e.g., Cronin, 2000) and evaluation theory (e.g., Narin, Olivastro & Stevens, 1994). Within the field of bibliometrics, there have been discussions of theory (e.g., *citationology*, Garfield, 1998), metatheory (e.g., *moral and political economy*; *structuration*; Cronin, 1998), and numerous references to methodologies. Bibliometric methods include such approaches as citation analysis, co-citation coupling, bibliographic coupling and coword analysis. The range of foci in bibliometric studies extends from macro levels examinations related to science policy to micro level examinations of the scholarship of individuals (e.g., Narin, Olivastro & Stevens, 1994). Common quantitative outcomes in bibliometrics are expressed in a number of laws, such as Bradford's Law of Scattering, Garfield's Constant, Garfield's Law of Concentration, Lotka's Law and Zipf's Law (Garfield, 1998). Bibliometrics have been used outside of social work in a range of areas including agriculture, the sciences, library and information sciences, medicine, social sciences, and technology (Sellen, 1993). In addition to numerous books on the subjects, there are a variety of journals related to this topical area including: *Cybermetrics: International Journal of Scientometrics, Informetrics and Bibliometrics*; *Information Processing & Management*; *Journal of the American Society for Information Science* (after 2000 titled *Journal of the American Society for Information Science and Technology*); *Journal of Documentation*; *Journal of the Medical Library Association*; *Library Collections, Acquisitions, and Technical Services*; *Scientometrics* and *Social Studies of Science*.

*Citation analysis*, a component of bibliometrics, focuses on the quantitative assessment of citation patterns in a body of literature. Citation analyses depend on citation indexes. Garfield noted:

> The concept of citation indexing is simple. Almost all the papers, reviews, corrections, and correspondence published in scientific journals contain citations. These cite . . . documents that support, provide precedent for, illustrate, or elaborate on what the author has to say. Citations are the formal, explicit linkages between papers that have particular points in common. A citation index is built around these linkages. (1979, p. 1)

Forms of citation indexing have been used since the 12th century (Wouters, 2000). More specific to the focus of this paper, citations have long been recognized as a potentially valid, although imperfect, measure of a scientist's impact (e.g., Myers, 1970; Oppenheim, 1997). In the past decade, citation analysis has been extended to the murkier world of the web with the advent of '*sitation analysis*' which is the analysis of the linkages between web sites (e.g., Rousseau, 1997).

Given the increasing number of publications covering bibliometrics in social work, it seemed to be an appropriate time to summarize that scholarship. This paper will therefore present a selective review of this area. In order to provide the reader with some methodological background with which they may approach the review more critically, a summary of critiques of bibliometric methods is presented first.

Both pros and cons have been raised regarding the use of bibliometrics both inside and outside of social work (e.g., Baker, 1990; 1991; 1992a; Borgman & Furner, 2002; Cnaan, Caputo & Shmuely, 1994; Cole, 2000; Cole & Cole, 1971; Garfield, 1997; Jones, 1999; Kirk, 1984; Kostoff, 2002; Krueger, 1993; Lindsey, 1978a; 1980; 1982; 1989; MacRoberts & MacRoberts, 1989; 1992; Plomp, 1990; Phelan, 1999; Porter, 1977; von Ungern-Sternberg, 2000). Many of these are detailed in Table 1. This list of disadvantages might cause a reader to think bibliometrics are a crude tool at best. For instance, MacRoberts and MacRoberts (1989) argued that until citation analysis received much more careful examination of the theories and assumptions upon which it is based, any findings from using this method would have to be considered very tentative. Lindsey (1989) asks if citation studies are "measuring what is measurable rather than what is valid" (p. 200) and Krueger (1993), in part, calls for a moratorium on the publication of studies that rank social work programs based on publication and citation counts.

Meinert (1993) responded to Krueger suggesting that it might be more productive to critically review and attempt to improve bibliometric methods. We agree with Meinert. Any research area worthy of investigation needs to have its methods continuously and critically reviewed. Research methods can take time to develop and they may be less than optimally applied during the development period (as well as afterward). Further, a number of these criticisms focus on inter-institutional comparisons. Bibliometrics has applications beyond studies that rank social work programs. We have suggested elsewhere (as have others) that bibliometrics could be used as a decision-making aid in academic hiring, reappointment, tenure and promotion decisions, as well as for descriptions of larger aggregations of scholarship such as journals. In general, one should

TABLE 1. Selected potential advantages and disadvantages of bibliometric analyses that have been noted in the literature.

| Advantages | Disadvantages |
| --- | --- |
| 1] Bibliometric methods facilitate examination of large data sets. | 1] Citation analyses may encounter measurement and technical problems including: spelling; name changes; homonyms; synonyms; clerical errors; changes in citation databases over time; language biases; problems with the journal impact factor. |
| 2] Bibliometric analyses can facilitate decision making regarding institutions (e.g., research funding). | 2] Sampling problems such as: some studies that have focused on a small selection of journals; non-article scholarship is ignored; and databases such as SSCI may not cover all the relevant journals or all of the volumes of journals that are included in the database. Journal coverage in the database may fluctuate over time. |
| 3] Bibliometric analyses can facilitate decision making regarding organizational issues (e.g., library collections). | 3] Citations may not be equivalent and the types of citations vary. Citations can occur for non-scientific reasons. They may not be positive and/or central to the issue being discussed. Authors may be more likely to reference work that: is indexed in more commonly used databases; is more easily available to them; is written in the language they speak; is newer; is a popular fad or trend; etc. |
| 4] Bibliometric analyses can facilitate decision making about individuals (e.g., hiring, reappointment, tenure, and promotion decisions) and by individuals (e.g., choice of publication outlets). | 4] Authors may be referencing themselves or colleagues and thereby inflating citation rates (self-citation). Similarly, authors might inappropriately cite friends, colleagues, mentors or editors of the journal. |
| 5] Bibliometrics can facilitate examination of the sociology of science (e.g., invisible colleges). | 5] Referencing patterns can vary across fields, nations, time period studied or publications. |
| 6] Bibliometrics can facilitate examination of trends in subject areas. | 6] Authors may be citing work that is incorrect, not citing the best work, not correctly citing satisfactory work or may be failing to cite work that influenced them. |

TABLE 1 (continued)

| Advantages | Disadvantages |
|---|---|
| 7] Bibliometrics can facilitate examination of trends within individual or sets of journals. | 7] Informal influences such as discussions with colleagues are ignored (acknowledgements and personal communications citations are not credited to the target individual in citation counts). |
| 8] Citations are measured on a ratio level scale (although the conceptual meaning of units may vary). | 8] Quality (and components of quality such as morals and ethics) is an important factor not necessarily captured by quantity of publication or number of citations. |
| 9] Scholars should be motivated to cite others work appropriately, as they are always at risk for exposure for doing otherwise. | 9] Citations are not measured on an interval level scale. |
| 10] Citation counts are less susceptible to manipulation by authors than publication counts. | 10] Citation analysis may be biased against high quality work that is published in very specialized journals that are read by relatively few scholars. |
| 11] Citations are a relatively reliable indicator. | 11] Citation analysis may not reflect the impact of unpublished scientific work or the impact a journal or article has on professionals who are reading it (but not writing and citing it). |
| 12] There is evidence supporting citations as a valid indicator of impact. | 13] Multiple authorship makes determination of appropriate authorship credit difficult. |
|  | 14] Skewed distributions (many do not publish) are often present which may cause problems of interpretation. |
|  | 15] The publication process is biased (e.g., towards dominant paradigms) and citation analysis is biased towards logical positivism. |
|  | 16] The submission to publication time lag may bias some studies. |
|  | 17] Publication analyses that are based on self-report surveys have the typical array of problems. |
|  | 18] Disadvantages specifically noted regarding studies involving social work faculty include issues such as: faculty demographic characteristics (e.g., age, level of turnover) that may impact results in organization focused studies depending on the time period studied; publication can be less than half of social work faculty's workload; citation counts may be biased against applied scientists; variation in publication practices (e.g., analyses are biased against programs that have heavier teaching loads and less support for research and writing); the relative rankings for schools are difficult to interpret. |

remember the Institute for Scientific Information's (ISI) suggestions for interpretation in citation analysis. These recommendations merit summation:

1. Compare like with like: scientists or papers in the same field and papers of the same vintage, since different fields exhibit different average rates of citations and older papers have more time to collect citations than younger papers.
2. Multiple measures (number papers, citations, cites/paper, percent cited vs. uncited) and large datasets are superior to single, thin ones.
3. Relative measures should be used, not merely absolute scores (such as setting citation counts relative to appropriate baseline, or average, scores).
4. Sometimes the area of research is not adequately surveyed by the database examined, in which case the measures will not be robust and could be misleading.
5. And, most important, that these methods should be used as supplement and not as replacement for careful consideration by informed peers or experts (ISI, 2003, p. 1).

The reader should keep these recommendations in mind while reading this article as well as other applications of bibliometrics in social work, in order to maximize the probability of arriving at valid conclusions.

## BIBLIOMETRICS IN SOCIAL WORK

Within social work, the productivity and impact of individuals and academic institutions has been examined using citation analysis. These are the focus of this paper and will be examined in the next sections. Bibliometric approaches have been used in other ways in social work. These include examination of: the production of books and dissertations in social work over time (Baker, 1991); evolving issues related to the Danish Welfare State (Wormell, 2000a; 2000b); the pattern of citations

*8*  *BIBLIOMETRICS IN SOCIAL WORK*

to articles published in drug and alcohol journals (Howard & Howard, 1992) the social work holdings of libraries (Jones & Jones, 1986); the relative importance of journals in social work (Williams, 2001); the impact of a social work journal over a decade (Rosenberg, Holden & Barker, 2005) the relationships among journals in the social work journal network (Baker, 1992b); the interaction of social work and other fields (Cheung, 1990); the use of social science literature in social work journals (Bush, Epstein & Sainz, 1997); the use of citations to contrast rapid assessment instruments (McMurty, Rose & Cisler, 2003); the relationship of citations to reputation as a social work researcher (Rothman, Kirk & Knapp, 2003); and the use of bibliometrics in academic employment decisions (Holden, Rosenberg & Barker, 2005).

## *Quantity*

Perhaps the most basic approach in bibliometrics is to calculate the number of publications by some individual or group. Table 2 details research on the quantity of scholarship of social workers. The reader should be aware that some of these study reports overlap. That is the same data (e.g., articles for a particular time period) may be included in more than one study. While the purposes of the citation analyses in Table 2 vary, we focused on findings relevant to the quantity of journal articles published by social workers. Unrelated findings from these studies have been omitted. The studies reviewed herewith include descriptions of the quantity of publications by: social work doctoral graduates; editorial board members; highly successful authors; schools of social work; and social work faculty in general, as well as faculty subgroups (e.g., females/males, African-Americans). Productivity statistics are provided for the reader and these calculations result from averaging the number of publications over a period of time. For instance, a faculty member who publishes one article every three years would have a yearly productivity rate of .33.

It should also be noted that the data source for a number of studies is the *Social Science Citation Index* (SSCI). SSCI is one of three databases

TABLE 2. Studies estimating the quantity of publication of social work scholars.

| Authors/Year | Sample | Data source | Productivity statistic | Findings |
|---|---|---|---|---|
| Lindsey (1976) | $N$ = 323 Editorial board members of psychology, social work and sociology journals. | Various abstracts (e.g., Psychological Abstracts) | Adjusted total articles published (during time periods which varied depending on the databases used). | Psychology editorial board members had the highest mean number of adjusted total articles (13.0) followed by sociology (8.1) and social work (1.0). |
| Kroll, H. W. (1976) | $N$ = 683 articles by social work faculty members in four social work journals. | Four social work journals | Number of articles in these journals during the 1965-74 period. Appears from report to be equal credit proportional counts for institutions. | Positively skewed productivity. The University of Chicago, Columbia University and the University of California: Berkeley were the most productive schools. |
| Kirk, Wasserstrum & Miller (1977) | Survey of all US and Canadian graduate programs. 32% of all schools responded describing a total n of 76 faculty members being reviewed for tenure or promotion during the 1974-75 academic year. | Mailed survey | Number of articles in refereed journals. | Positively skewed productivity. 33% had not published an article, 10% published 10 articles or more. Mean n of articles = 3.7. |
| Rosen (1979) | $N$ = 3081% of the PhD graduates from Washington University during the 6/70-5/78 period. | Mailed survey & academic records | Total productivity index. Output weighted as follows: authored books = 5; edited books = 2.5; article, chapter, monograph = 2; unpublished conference presentation = 1.25; unpublished paper = 1. Single, first and second listed authors given full weight, all other authors .5 of the weight. | Positively skewed productivity. Total productivity index: min - max: 2.0 - 102.0, $M$ = 22.8 ($SD$ = 24.4). |

TABLE 2 (continued)

| Authors/Year | Sample | Data source | Productivity statistic | Findings |
|---|---|---|---|---|
| Jayaratne (1979) | N = 79 schools Articles by social work faculty members | Five social work journals | Normal count. n of articles per faculty member for the 1972-76 period[1] | Positively skewed productivity. Mean n of .29 articles per faculty member in the selected journals for the period. |
| Kirk & Rosenblatt (1980) | N = 9,967 articles All articles in these journals | Five social work journals | Sex distribution of authors for the 1934-77 period. | Proportion of male authors for the period was .45. |
| McNeece (1981) | N = 97 50.5% response rate to a randomly selected list of US MSW program faculty | Mailed survey | N of articles in refereed journals for 1978 | Positively skewed productivity distribution–56% of the respondents did not publish an article in 1978. Mean n of articles = 876) |
| Council on Social Work Education (CSWE, 1983-2000) | varies | Yearly survey of CSWE accredited programs for the publication *Statistics on Social Work Education in the United States* | Average number of articles in the most recent 12 month period in refereed journals. The authors of these reports caution the reader to be wary of this data, because of missing data and their inability to know how many respondents adjusted the total number of reported publications for multiple authorship as instructed (e.g., if two colleagues co-authored an article each would receive .5 of a credit). | When article productivity distribution reported it was positively skewed. Average numbers of faculty member articles were: .39 (83); .38 (84); .41 (85); .35 (86); .46 (87); .43 (88); .42 (89); .38 (90); .30 (91); .30 (92); .28 (93); .26 (94); .29 (95); .29 (96); .31 (97); .27 (98); .32 (99); .26 (00). |
| Grinnell & Royer (1983) | N = 10,416 Full length articles | Sixteen social work journals for the | Proportion of articles published by senior/sole authors' affiliation during the life of the journal (initial publication– 1/1/79 period). | University affiliated senior/sole authors published the largest proportion of articles (41.5%) followed by those affiliated with government (27.1%) and private agencies (24.3%) |

| Kirk & Rosenblatt (1984) | $N$ = 593 social work faculty $N$ = 439 articles by them. | Sixteen social work journals | Equal credit proportional count and productivity ratio (% of articles / % of faculty), for articles published during the 1977-79 period. | Compared men and women at five faculty ranks. Males produced greater percentage of articles at all five. |
|---|---|---|---|---|
| Abbott (1985) | $N$ = 175 50% response rate from a random sample of 350 doctoral program graduates | Mailed survey & *Social Science Citation Index* | $N$ of articles in refereed social work journals on which the respondent was the first or second author during two periods (graduation (1960-74)/1975 & 1976-1981). | Positively skewed productivity distributions. Respondents published a annual mean of .5 articles per year during the graduation/1975 period and .25 articles per year during the 1976-81 period. |
| Fox & Faver (1985) | $N$ = 300 Subset of the 64% response rate to a random survey of faculty in 44 US graduate social work programs. | Mailed survey | $N$ of journal articles in the two years prior to the study | Positively skewed productivity distributions. Men published slightly more articles during the period than women (2.1 vs. 1.63, $p < .1$). |
| Robbins, Corcoran, Hepler & Magner (1985) | $N$ = 286 46% response rate to a randomly distributed survey of undergraduate and graduate accredited programs in the US. | Mailed survey | $N$ of single and joint authored articles during the 1972-82 time period. | Positively skewed productivity distributions. Assistant, associate and full professors produced .77, 2.1 and 4.0 single authored articles respectively. Assistant, associate and full professors produced .90, 1.61 and 2.05 jointly authored articles respectively. |
| Smith, Baker, Campbell & Cunningham (1985) | $N$ = 128 Faculty from a mixed method approach with an initial random sample from 299 accredited US social work programs | Mailed survey | Recent and career productivity. n of articles published and accepted for publication during 1980-82 period and for entire career. | Positively skewed productivity distribution for 1980-82. |

TABLE 2 (continued)

| Authors/Year | Sample | Data source | Productivity statistic | Findings |
|---|---|---|---|---|
| Thyer & Bentley (1986) | All articles in these journals | Six social work journals | Normal count. Number of times a school's faculty member was listed as an author on a journal article during the 1979-83 period. | Positively skewed productivity distribution. University of Wisconsin-Madison faculty appeared most frequently in this set of journals during the 1979-83 period. |
| Rubin & Powell (1987) | $N = 1,002$ FT faculty members in CSWE accredited graduate programs with more than 50% teaching responsibilities and no administrative position | CSWE Annual Statistics (self/school-report) | Normal count. $n$ of articles per faculty member for 1983 & 1984. | Replicated analyses for 1984 for the significant findings in the 1983 data. Only significant result replicated was that female professors with non-social work doctorates published more book chapters than their counterparts. |
| Corcoran & Kirk (1990) | All articles authored by social work faculty in these journals. | Sixteen social work journals for the 1977-82 period & a subset of seven academic social work journals for the 1977-87 period. | Normal count. $n$ of articles in three types of journals during two time periods (1977-82; 1977-87). | Positively skewed productivity distributions. Average faculty member produced .39 academic journal articles, .06 agency journal articles and .16 mixed journal articles for the 1977-82 period. For the 1977-87 period, the average faculty member produced .79 articles in academic journals. |
| Schiele (1991) | $N = 290$ Usable response rate = 48.7%. African-American faculty in CSWE preaccredited & accredited programs in 1989-90 | Two mailed surveys. | $n$ of articles published during career. | Positively skewed productivity distribution. Mean n of articles during career was 1.84 in social work journals and 1.85 in non-social work journals. |

| | | | | |
|---|---|---|---|---|
| Baker & Wilson (1992) | $N = 284$<br>Mixed (random/100%) sample of doctoral graduates from 30 social work programs (1970-80) identified by Social Work Abstracts/Social Work Research & Abstracts | Source index of *Social Science Citation Index* | $n$ of articles during the graduation and the 6 subsequent years. | Positively skewed productivity distribution. 50% of the sample had not published an article that appeared in the SSCI database. Minimum–maximum: 0 - 13 articles. $M = 1.34$ ($SD = 1.98$) for the 7 year period and an annual mean productivity of .19 articles. |
| Green, Hutchison & Sar (1992) | $N = 1548$<br>56% response rate subsequently adjusted to the n of 1548. Social work doctoral program graduates[2] from the 1960-88 period | Mailed survey | Normal count. $n$ of articles since receiving the doctorate. | Positively skewed productivity distributions. Average graduate published 3.44 articles in social work and 3.40 articles in non social work journals during their career. |
| Mokau, Hull & Burkett (1993) | $N = 85$<br>43% response rate to random sample of 200 undergraduate CSWE accredited program directors | Mailed survey | Number of articles in prior 12 months | Positively skewed productivity distribution. 71% of the respondents did not publish an article in the prior 12 months. Mean $n$ of publications = .26 |

TABLE 2 (continued)

| Authors/Year | Sample | Data source | Productivity statistic | Findings |
|---|---|---|---|---|
| Green & Bentley (1994) (c.f., Green & Secret, 1996) | $N = 202$ "most successful" from a group of 3,423 authors who had published in a set of 18 social work journals during the 1980's (useable response rate of 81%) | Mailed survey | Professional journal articles published during entire career. | Positively skewed productivity distribution. 88.1% of sample were full time faculty. Number of articles for their career: min-max: 5-145, $M = 26.47$ ($SD = 18.13$). Mean yearly rate of 2.08. |
| Hull & Johnston (1994) | $N = 167$ Baccalaureate faculty who had published in the seven journals. | Seven social work journals. | Normal count. $n$ of articles during the 1985-mid 1991 period. | Positively skewed productivity distribution. Among those that did publish, the mean $n$ of publications was 1.49 for the 6.5 year period. |
| Thyer, Boynton, Bennis & Levine (1994) | All regular articles in these journals | Six social work journals | Normal count. Number of times a school's faculty member was listed as an author on a journal article during the 1984-88 period. | Positively skewed productivity distribution. University of Michigan faculty appeared most frequently in this set of journals during the 1984-88 period. |
| Johnson & Hull, (1995) | $N = 198$ Undergraduate faculty in CSWE accredited programs in the 1988-92 period (response rate not reported). | Mailed survey | Devised scoring system for multiple authorship, but focus here is the n of articles during the 1988-92 period. | Positively skewed productivity distribution. Total of 240 articles; 1.21 per faculty member for an annual average rate of .24 articles. |

| Study | Sample | Source | Method | Findings |
|---|---|---|---|---|
| Ligon, Thyer & Dixon (1995) | $N$ = 1480 authors from 245 academic institutions | Six social work journals | Normal count. Number of times a school's faculty member was listed as an author on a journal article during the 1989-93 period. | Positively skewed productivity distribution. University of Maryland at Baltimore faculty appeared most frequently in this set of journals during the 1989-93 period. |
| Pardeck, Chung, & Murphy (1995) | $N$ = 123 editorial board members & 106 guest reviewers from "core" social work journals. | Social Science Citation Index & Psychological Abstracts | Total $N$ of articles published by editorial board members and guest reviewers that were listed in Psychological Abstracts during 1987-90. | Positively skewed productivity distribution. The median number of articles published for both editorial board members and guest reviewers was 1 or less for the 1987-1990 period. |
| Green, Baskind & Conklin (1995)[3] (c.f., Green, Baskind, Best & Boyd, 1997) | $N$ = 1,084 Full time US social work doctoral faculty in the 1/90-9/93 period | Mailed surveys to obtain list of faculty. Social Science Citation Index | Combined normal & straight count. Number of articles published during 1990-93 period | Positively skewed productivity distribution. Average faculty member published 1.25 articles during the period. |
| Green (1998) | $N$ = 535 Full time US social work MSW/PhD faculty in 1994 | Mailed survey | No multiple authorship adjustment. $N$ of journals submitted and accepted or published by 5/1/95 in a group 55 social work journals. | Positively skewed productivity distribution–28.9% of these faculty did not submit an article during 1994. Faculty submitted an average of 2.11 articles during 1994. |

TABLE 2 (continued)

| Authors/Year | Sample | Data source | Productivity statistic | Findings |
|---|---|---|---|---|
| Seaberg (1998) | $N = 149$ Mixed method from an initial stratified random sample of 40 accredited graduate social work programs. 49% response rate from faculty members at final step. | Mailed survey | $n$ of peer reviewed articles over a two year period. | Positively skewed productivity distribution. Mean n of articles = 1.5 per year (1.8 for "active" scholars). |
| Pardeck & Meinert (1999a) | $N = 55$ Editorial board members and consulting editors of *Social Work* in 1/96 | *Psychological Abstracts, Social Work Abstracts, Sociological Abstracts, and the Social Science Citation Index* | Total $N$ of articles published by editorial board members and consulting editors during 1990-95 (and listed in these sources). | For the 1990-1995 period, 50% of the editorial board members and 19% of the consulting editors did not publish an article that appeared in the first three of these data sources. |
| Green, Kvarfordt & Hayden (2001)[3] | $N = 45$ Social work faculties' publications during the 1994-97 period. | *Social Science Citation Index* | Combined normal & straight count. Number of articles published during 1994-97 period. | Positively skewed productivity distribution. Columbia University faculty had the highest total productivity (unadjusted for faculty size). |
| Ligon & Thyer (2001) | $N = 1093$ articles | Six social work journals | Normal count. Number of times a school's faculty member was listed as an author on a journal article during the 1994-98 period. | Positively skewed productivity distribution. Columbia University faculty appeared most frequently in this set of journals during the 1994-98 period. |

| Green, Baskind & Bellin (2002)[3] | $N = 61$ Social work faculties | *Social Science Citation Index* | Combined normal & straight count. Number of articles published during the 1990-99 period. | Positively skewed productivity distribution overall for the decade. Total $n$ of articles published by the 61 schools during the period was 4,406 (min-max: 3-259, $M = 72.23$). There was a trend over the decade with mean yearly rates of 6.61 (1990-93); 7.43 (1994-97); 8.02 (1998-99). |
|---|---|---|---|---|
| Pardeck (2002) | $N = 10$ Psychology and social work journal editors | *PsychInfo* and the *Social Science Citation Index* | Number of articles published from 1992 through 6/01 that were covered in *PsychInfo*. | Social work editorial board members published an average of 3.4 during the 1992 through 6/01 period, whereas psychology board members published an average of 24.4 articles. |

Note: *Adjusted total articles*–each article is divided by the number of authors and then summed. *Normal counts (aka whole counts)*–multiple individuals receive full credit for a single article. *Straight counts–give all credit to the first author. Equal credit proportional counts– Co-authors receive equal credit proportions (e.g., three authors each receive .333). Combined normal & straight count* (Green, Baskind & Conklin, 1995)–when co-authors were on same faculty only the first (or only one credit granted to that faculty) was credited so that schools received only one credit per article, though multiple schools could each receive credit for publication (c.f., Cronin & Overfelt, 1994).
1. A second time period was included in another aspect of this study.
2. Included interdisciplinary doctorates from Brandeis who did not have masters in social work.
3. The same data is used for elements of these studies as they were all part of the Virginia Commonwealth University *Doctoral Faculty Decade Publication Project.*

*18* BIBLIOMETRICS IN SOCIAL WORK

that comprise the Web of Science (WoS) available from Thomson's Institute for Scientific Information (*http://isi4.isiknowledge.com/portal. cgi*). Thomson claimed that in January 2004, SSCI covered over 1700 social science journals and the three WoS databases combined covered approximately 8500 journals.

In terms of quantity of publications, the studies found in Table 2 generally support the notion that social work scholars publish in both social work and non-social work journals. Many of these studies also reveal that a substantial proportion of faculty never or rarely publish, while a much smaller subset of faculty are relatively prolific. This finding appears to coincide with *Lotka's Law of Scientific Productivity of Authors*. Lotka's law states that "the number (of authors) making $n$ contributions is about $1/n^2$ of those making one; and the proportion of all contributors that make a single contribution, is about 60%" (Twining, 2002). Therefore, the relative percentages of the authors contributing $n$ articles within an analysis should be (approximately): 60% of authors would have published 1 article; 25% would have published 2 articles; 11% would have published 3 articles and so on (this is obviously a rough approximation given that the proportions exceed 100%). While insufficient data was available in most of these studies to calculate comparable statistics, the rough form of positive skew represented by Lotka's Law was observed. For instance, Hull and Johnston (1994) found that in the seven journals they studied for the 1985-1991 period, approximately 9% ($n = 167$) of undergraduate faculty published an article. Of those 167 who published, 73% published one article. A positively skewed productivity distribution appears at the academic organization level as well with approximately 20% of the doctoral faculties producing 44% of the articles in one major study (Green, Baskind & Bellin, 2002).

It is also worth noting that differences in sampling (e.g., time periods, journals, schools) and operational definitions (what is a "publication") make other comparisons difficult. It is clear that research on practitioner publication is much more rare than research on faculty publication. While practitioners were included in some of these studies, analysis of them as a subgroup was not clearly executed. For instance, studies of social work doctoral program graduates likely included current and past faculty.

## *Impact*

How should one think about the quantity of scholarship versus the impact of scholarship? Should one be emphasized over the other or should one seek a relatively balanced combination? The Coles (Cole & Cole, 1967) grappled with this issue in their examination of physicists by describing existing patterns of publications. They proposed four rough types: the prolific physicist (high quantity, high quality), the mass producer, the perfectionist and the silent physicist (low quantity, low quality). Lindsey (1978b) proposed the *corrected quality ratio*, which combined the n of publications and n of citations (using a variety of adjustments, but it has not been used frequently (Glanzel & Moed, 2002). Note that throughout our studies, the focus is on impact rather than 'quality' which is a more difficult to define construct that has led to criticisms of bibliometrics in the past (Phelan, 1999). Although we raise the question of what is the desired mix of quantity and impact, a serious discussion is beyond the scope of this article.

In the narrative review provided below, we focus on impact (operationalized as citations to journal articles), as *an* indicator of the quality of a scholar's work (c.f., Garfield, 1996; Narin, Olivastro & Stevens, 1994). The early assumption that citations were equivalent to quality has often been critiqued. Lindsey (1989) discusses these limitations and uses the term contribution at one point, which also seems less problematic than quality. Kostoff (2002) notes: "[t]he assumption is then made that documents with higher relative numbers of citation counts have more impact than those with lower citation counts, and are of higher quality from a citation metric perspective" (p. 50). Our view is that impact is a more neutral term than quality or contribution and that impact and quality are imperfectly correlated. For instance, (to echo Lindsey's (1989) point about work outside the dominant paradigm) a very high quality article may be infrequently cited because the author has chosen a topic that is of little interest to colleagues during the years subsequent to

## BIBLIOMETRICS IN SOCIAL WORK

its publication. While some of the following studies we discus below were included in Table 2 if they reported quantity data, we return to them here because the authors also reported citation analyses.

In the 1970s, Lindsey published a series of seminal pieces that set a standard for bibliometrics in social work. For instance, he examined a proportional, stratified, random sample of journal articles from the sciences (biochemistry) and the social sciences (economics, psychiatry, psychology, social work and sociology) published in 1970 (Lindsey, 1978a). He found that social work articles had fewer references to prior work than the other surveyed fields. In terms of citations to the articles (during the 1970-1976 period), the distribution of citations was positively skewed in all fields and social work had the lowest overall mean and median numbers of citations. Lindsey noted: "In all of the fields, 10 percent of the papers attracted 42 to 49 percent of the citations. Most of the papers that are published are rarely, if ever, used by future investigators" (p. 92).

*Impact of editors.* One line of subsequent research stemmed from Lindsey's (1976; c.f., Lindsey, 1978a, Ch. 4) contrast of the productivity of psychology, social work and social work journal editorial board members. Utilizing various citation related indicators as measures of quality, Lindsey concluded that social work editorial board members produced less and lower quality scholarship. Pardeck et al. (1991) partially replicated Lindsey's studies from the mid- to late-1970s and contrasted five social work and five psychology journal editorial boards. They used the number of times each editorial board member was cited (when they were the first author) in the SSCI in 1989 as the outcome and found that psychology editorial board members were cited more frequently in 1989. The re-analysis of this data (Pardeck, 1992a) was published in *Research on Social Work Practice* along with a series of commentaries (Epstein, 1992; Fortune, 1992; Gillespie & Khinduka, 1992; Hopps, 1992; Lindsey, 1992; Reamer, 1992; Schuerman, 1992) and a reply from Pardeck (1992b). The finding that journal editorial board members in psychology were cited more frequently than those in social work was replicated in the re-analysis. Conceptual and methodological issues were framed as concerns in many of the commentaries.

Responding in part to commentators' criticisms, Pardeck, Chung and Murphy (1995) reported a replication and extension of Pardeck and Lindsey's earlier work. Looking at editorial board members and guest reviewers for six core social work journals for the 1987-90 period, they found that the median number of articles published ranged from 0 to 1 (depending on the journal). During this period, the percentage of board members and reviewers who were cited three times or less during the four year period ranged from 0 to 53% across the six journals. These findings may underestimate editorial board impact because citations were only counted when the board member/reviewer was the first or sole author and self-citations were not included. Multiple authorship and self citation are potential problems in bibliometrics and although the approach used in this study has been employed in other studies, we have suggested elsewhere that this practice may not be optimal (Holden, Rosenberg & Barker, 2005).

These editorial board scholarship analyses were replicated again, when Pardeck and Meinart (1999a) examined the editorial board and consulting editors of *Social Work*. Productivity (articles) and impact (citations) for the 1990-95 period were analyzed. In terms of productivity, 50% of the editorial board and 19.1% of the consulting editors did not publish an article that the authors could uncover in their search of three sources (*Social Work Abstracts*, *Sociological Abstracts* and *Psychological Abstracts*). In terms of impact, 50% of the editorial board and 23.4% of the consulting editors fell in the category of 0-3 citations during the six years. As in the first version of this publication, there were a series of responses (Browning & Winchester, 1999; Epstein, 1999; Ginsberg, 1999; Karger, 1999; Kreuger, 1999; Lindsey, 1999; Midgley, 1999; Reamer, 1999) and a response to these responses (Pardeck & Meinart, 1999b). In that response, Pardeck and Meinart note that:

> Within the field of social work, the worship of diversity may have overshadowed the importance of social work as the features of science have been devalued. In all activities, we insist on casting the widest inclusionary net and are fearful of leaving out a group; yet

at the same time, we do not exhibit the same degree of insistence that scientific merit be included. (p. 123)

Pardeck's (2002) most recent research entailed contrasting the productivity of the editors of five major psychology with five major social work journals. During the 1992 through June 2001 period, the psychology editors published 24.4 articles on average ($SD$ = 9.5), whereas the social work editors published 3.4 articles on average ($SD$ = 4.22; $M$ = .36 articles per year, per editor). In terms of citations (the same restriction to sole or first authors as noted above), psychology editors were cited 76.8 times on average during a five year period (1995-99), while social work editors were cited 9.28 times ($M$ = 1.86 times per year, per editor).

These results for social work editors are disquieting (c.f., Lindsey, 1999 for similar preliminary results regarding endowed chairs in social work). Even with acquiescence to the view that more is required of an editor than being a prolific scholar (e.g., Reamer, 1999), the role of editor is a self-selected one that hinges on, presumably at least in part, a quest for knowledge, scholarship and writing. In depth discussion of the reasons for this consistent and dramatic differentiation is beyond the scope of this article but root causes are likely many. As one of our reviewers alluded to, is this simply a difference in publication and citation norms of the two fields (e.g., ISI, 2003; Najman & Hewitt, 2003)? Lindsey (1991) has noted the related issue that there seem to be differences between 'academic' and 'practice' fields in the amounts of citations received (Lindsey, 1991). Other questions could be raised. Are academic institutions providing enough support for journal editors in social work? Is editing a social work journal different than editing journals in other fields (i.e., more onerous)? These issues are worthy of empirical investigation and discussion. Despite the need for further research in this area, Lindsey's and Pardeck's research has illuminated and maintained a focus on the situation that may have already (or may in the future) increased the presence of active scholars on editorial boards in social work.

A related issue is the quality of peer review. It has seemed clear for some time that the peer review process in social work can be problematic (c.f., Lindsey, 1978c; 1988; 1991; 1999; Pardeck & Meinart, 1999b). We assume that this is, in part, due to a failure on the part of academics to teach students to carry out this professional responsibility. Lindsey's and Pardeck's findings may be an additional component of the explanation of this problem. If one is not taught how to perform constructive peer review, and one rarely publishes (thereby having both positive and negative models of the peer review process), then the likelihood that one would produce strong reviews is reduced. Regardless, higher quality peer review is so important to the profession that it deserves ever more serious attention by editors, scholars and faculty responsible for the design of doctoral curricula.

*Impact of journals.* Lindsey and Kirk (1992) used the impact factor score (IFS) to contrast the impact of social work journals. The IFS was developed by Garfield and Sher in the early 1960s (Garfield, 1999). A journal's IFS is computed by "dividing the number of citations in year 3 to any items published in the journal in years 1 and 2 by the number of substantive articles published in that journal in years 1 and 2" (Saha, Saint & Christakis, 2003, p. 43). Lindsey and Kirk compared social work journals' IFSs and found that of the core social work journals, *Social Work* (SW) had the highest IFS during the 1981-89 period (mean = .70). These authors suggest that such findings may be due in part to the vast differentials in the distribution of SW relative to specialty journals, and others have reported a strong positive correlation ($r = .68$) between journal citation rates and the size of the journals' circulation (Howard & Howard, 1992). With bibliometric indicators, as with any indicator in the social sciences, one needs to be cautious about regarding the psychometric properties of the indicator. IFSs have received support as an indicator of journal quality (Christenson & Sigelman, 1985; Saha, Saint & Christakis, 2003), although they have also been critiqued regarding a number of issues (e.g., Frank, 2003; Garfield, 1996; Glanzel & Moed, 2002). For instance, within social work, Furr (1995) reported findings suggesting that the IFS may not reflect impact within the journal's discipline, as opposed to across disciplines (as they are currently computed).

*Impact of authors in social work journals.* Dumas, Logan and Finley (1993) studied citations to articles published in the *British Journal of Social Work* (BJSW) and *Social Work* (SW) during the 1984-91 period and described the highly cited articles and subject categories for each journal. The most highly cited article in the BJSW had been cited 16 times during the period, whereas the most highly cited article in SW had been cited 29 times during the period. Eight articles from SW were cited 20 or more times. Conversely, there were 89 articles in the *British Journal of Social Work* and 231 articles in *Social Work* that had only been cited one time during the period. In terms of interpreting the differences in citations rates, Dumas, Logan and Finley suggest that the smaller number of articles in each issue of BJSW, along with its less frequent rate of publication should be considered. Differences in citation norms may also have been a factor.

*Impact of faculty.* In their 1992 paper, Klein and Bloom sought to help the profession reduce the level of subjectivity in tenure and promotion decisions. They reported four studies using citation analysis. In the first study of social work experts (authors in the *Encyclopedia of Social Work*), they found that in 1987 these experts averaged 9.4 citations per person, and among academics, full professors (13.7) were cited more than associate professors (7.6) and assistant professors (4.7). In their second study, Klein and Bloom found that the 99 deans and directors of CSWE accredited programs were cited an average of 2.9 times in 1987. In their third study of a convenience sample of four U.S. schools of social work, they found that full professors were cited more frequently, but that the rankings were mixed for associate and assistant professors. They also found generally lower average rates of citation for faculty in these four "major" schools compared to the expert and deans samples. In their fourth study of three individual faculty, Klein and Bloom employed statistics such as the write/cite index, lag time and persistence that allow for a more in-depth view of three scholars' work.

Subsequently, Bloom and Klein (1995) studied 344 faculty (333 for whom cites were found) from the top 13 schools in the Thyer and Bentley (1986) study. Overall, they found that 29.7% of these faculty had a publication listed in SSCI and that 76.6% of these faculty had been cited. The average rate of publication for these faculty was .56 and the average number of citations per faculty was 9.55 in 1992. Bloom and Klein combined three variables (average total journal articles published, proportion of all faculty members publishing, and average number of citations) to create a critical mass of scholarship score which they saw as a more comprehensive measure of an institution's scholarly productivity. The mean critical mass score in this sample of 13 schools was 2.49, which was exceeded by the University of California-Berkeley ($M = 11.58$), Columbia University ($M = 6.27$), Washington University ($M = 3.34$), the University of Wisconsin-Madison ($M = 3.26$) and the University of Washington-Seattle ($M = 2.78$).

In another study that contrasted psychologists with social workers, Thyer and Polk (1997) randomly selected 20 universities with doctoral programs and then obtained the names of full professors in the social work and psychology programs at these universities. Thyer and Polk determined the number of times that each of these full professors were cited in the SSCI during 1994. Given the positive skew of the citation distributions for each group, Thyer and Polk reported the median number of citations for the full professors, which was 19 for psychology and 4 for social work. More recently, Green and Hayden (2001) examined the number of published articles and citations for the ten most productive social work faculties during the 1990-1997 period. The average faculty member on these faculties published 4.4 articles during the period with those articles being cited 3.27 times on average (means were positively skewed by the University of California-Berkeley faculty). Perhaps most revealing was that non social work journal articles were much more frequently cited (4.22 times per non-social work vs. 1.69 times per social work article). For both of these studies, as with the inter-professional contrasts of journal editors reported above, the possibility of differing norms of citing behavior remains one possible, partial explanation of the results.

A small body of knowledge regarding the impact of social work scholarship has been evolving since Lindsey's 1978 work. The emerging picture seems to be that as a group, social work faculty were publishing regularly, although productivity is skewed, with a small group of authors responsible for a disproportionate share of the output. In terms of impact, we have preliminary evidence: that impact as measured by citations is similarly skewed with a small group of papers receiving most of the citations; that as one might expect, full professors tended to have higher rates of citation, as do deans and 'experts' in the field; and that social work faculty publications in non-social work journals were more likely to be cited.

Although less is known about the scholarship of practitioners as a group, some researchers have begun to study the topic (e.g., Bush, Epstein & Sainz, 1997; Rehr, Showers, Rosenberg & Blumenfield, 1998; Staudt, Dulmus & Bennett, 2003). Further investigation of the scholarship of practitioners is in order. As Rehr, Rosenberg, Showers and Blumenfield (1998) suggest, "[w]e need to learn, from practice writings, what concerns clinicians, and what they have examined" (p. 76).

Examination of practitioners' scholarship is but one possibility in an area that is ripe for exploration. Our group has explored the use of bibliometrics in academic employment decisions (Holden, Rosenberg & Barker, 2005) and the examination of the output of a core social work journal over the course of a decade (Rosenberg, Holden & Barker, 2005). These represent merely two among many possible lines of research.

## CONCLUSION

Like any other area of study, bibliometrics is in a process of evolution. To date, the field has provided us with some fascinating windows into the world of scholarship. As can be seen from the preceding review, social workers are publishing journal articles and these articles are having an impact. Yet, there is much to learn about these processes and outcomes. Although the methods of citation analyses have varied, over time more agreement about the best methods should emerge and estimates will become easier to interpret. Scholars are developing bibliometric methods and advocating for the development of databases such as the WoS. The prevailing views of citation analysis as a method appear to range from the relatively positive, such as the one you have encountered in this paper, to the relatively negative (e.g., MacRoberts & MacRoberts, 1989). Social workers should remember that both bibliometrics and scientometrics are subsumed under the general field of informetrics (Brookes, 1990). The evolution of easily accessible, full-text source materials opens up even more informetric research possibilities (c.f., Borgman & Furner, 2002).

In our view, it is too early to "go negative" on bibliometrics. In closing, we offer the simple maxim oft stated: Better data leads to better decisions. Better bibliographic data will lead to better understanding of, and decisions about, social work scholarship.

## REFERENCES

Abbott, A. A. (1985). Research productivity patterns of social work doctorates. *Social Work Research and Abstracts, 21, 3,* 11-17.

Baker, D. R. (1990). Citation analysis: A methodological review. *Social Work Research & Abstracts, 26,* 3-10.

Baker, D. R. (1991). On-line bibliometric analysis for researchers and educators. *Journal of Social Work Education, 27,* 41-47.

Baker, D. R. (1992a). Author responds. *Social Work Research & Abstracts, 28,* 4-5.

Baker, D. R. (1992b). A structural analysis of the social work journal network: 1985-1986. *Journal of Social Service Research, 15,* 153-168.

Baker, D. R. & Wilson, M. V. K. (1992). An evaluation of the scholarly productivity of doctoral graduates. *Journal of Social Work Education, 28,* 204-213.

Bar-Ilan, J. (2001). Data collection methods on the Web for informetric purposes–A review and analysis. *Scientometrics, 50, 1,* 7-32.

Black, P. E. (2002). Lotka's law. Retrieved 12/23/02 from: http://www.nist.gov/dads/HTML/lotkaslaw.html

Bloom, M. & Klein, W. C. (1995). Publications & citations: A study of faculty at leading schools of social work. *Journal of Social Work Education, 31,* 377-387.

Borgman, C. L. & Furner, J. (2002). Scholarly communication and bibliometrics. In B. Cronin (Ed.), *Annual Review of Information Science and Technology, 36* (pp. 3-72). Medford, NJ: Information Today.

## 28 BIBLIOMETRICS IN SOCIAL WORK

Brookes, B. C. (1990). Biblio-, sciento-, infor-metrics??? What are we talking about? In L. Egghe & R. Rosseau (Eds.), *Informetrics 89/90*. (pp. 31-44). Amsterdam: Elsevier.

Browning, J. & Winchester, N. (1999). Scholarship, inclusiveness, and *Social Work. Research on Social Work Practice, 9*, 113-4.

Bush, I., Epstein, I. & Sainz, A. (1997). The use of social science sources in social work practice journals: An application of citation analysis. *Social Work Research, 21, 1*, 45-56.

Cheung, K. M. (1990). Interdisciplinary relationships between social work and other disciplines: A citation study. *Social Work Research and Abstracts, 26, 3*, 23-9.

Christenson, J.A. & Sigelman, L. (1985). Accrediting knowledge: Journal stature and citation impact in social science. *Social Science Quarterly, 66*, 964-975

Cnaan, R. A., Caputo, R. K. & Shmuely, Y. (1994). Senior faculty perceptions of social work journals. *Journal of Social Work Education, 30*, 185-199.

Cole, J. R. (2000). A short history of the use of citations as a measure of the impact of scientific and scholarly work. In B. Cronin & H. B. Atkins (Eds.), *The Web of Knowledge: A Festchrift in Honor of Eugene Garfield*. (pp. 281-300). Medford, NY: Information Today.

Cole, J. & Cole, S. (1971). Measuring the quality of sociological research: Problems in the use of the *Science Citation Index. The American Sociologist, 6*, 23-29.

Cole, S. & Cole, J. (1967). Scientific output and recognition: A study of the reward system in science. *American Sociological Review, 32*, 377-390.

Corcoran, K. J. & Kirk, S. A. (1990). We're all number one: Academic productivity among schools of social work. *Journal of Social Work Education, 26*, 310-321.

Cronin, B. (1998). Metatheorizing citation. *Scientometrics, 43*, 45-55.

Cronin, B. (2000). Semiotics and evaluative bibliometrics. *Journal of Documentation, 56*, 440-453.

Cronin, B. & Overfelt, K. (1994). Citation-based auditing of academic performance. *Journal of the American Society for Information Science, 45, 2*, 61-72.

Dumas, T., Logan, E. & Finley, A. (1993). In focus: Using citation analysis and subject classification to identify and monitor trends within a discipline. In S. Bonzi (Ed.), *Proceedings of the 56th Annual Meeting of the American Society for Information Science*. (pp. 135-50). Medford, NJ: Learned Information, Inc.

Epstein, W. M. (1992). A response to Pardeck: Thump therapy for social work journals. *Research on Social Work Practice, 2*, 525-528.

Epstein, W. M. (1999). Of newsletters and scholarly journals. *Research on Social Work Practice, 9*, 111-112.

Fortune, A. E. (1992). More is not better–manuscript reviewer competence and citations: From the Past Editor-in-Chief of *Journal of Social Work Education. Research on Social Work Practice, 2*, 505-510.

Fox, M. F. & Faver, C. A. (1985). Men, women, and publication productivity: Patterns among social work academics. *Sociological Quarterly, 26*, 537-549.

Frank, M. (2003). Impact factors: Arbiter of excellence. *Journal of the American Medical Library Association, 91*, 4-6.

Franck, G. (2002). The scientific economy of attention: A novel approach to the collective rationality of science. *Scientometrics, 55, 1,* 3-26.

Fraser, M. W. (1994). Scholarship and research in social work: Emerging challenges. *Journal of Social Work Education, 30,* 252-266.

Furr, A. L. (1995). The relative influence of social work journals: Impact factors vs. core influence. *Journal of Social Work Education, 31,* 38-45.

Garfield, E. (1979). A conceptual view of citation indexing. In E. Garfield (Ed.), *Citation indexing–Its theory and application in science, technology and humanities.* (pp. 1-5). New York: John Wiley.

Garfield, E. (1996). How can impact factors be improved? *BMJ, 313, 7054,* 411-413.

Garfield, E. (1997). Validation of citation analysis. *Journal of the American Society for Information Science, 48,* 962-964.

Garfield, E. (1998). Random thoughts on citationology. Its theory and practice. *Scientometrics, 43,* 69-76.

Garfield, E. (1999). Journal impact factor: A brief review. *Canadian Medical Association Journal, 161,* 979-980.

Gastel, B. (2001). Assessing the impact of investigators' work: Beyond impact factors. *Canadian Journal of Anesthesia, 48,* 941-945.

Gillespie, D. F. & Khinduka, S. (1992). A response to Pardeck: From the Associate Editor and the Chair of the Editorial Board of the *Journal of Social Service Research. Research on Social Work Practice, 2,* 511-514.

Ginsberg, L. (1999). Reviewers, orthodoxy, and the passion to publish. *Research on Social Work Practice, 9,* 100-103.

Glanzel, W. & Moed, H. F. (2002). Journal impact measures in bibliometric research. *Scientometrics, 53, 2,* 171-193.

Green, R.G. (1998). Faculty rank, effort, and success: A study of publication in professional journals. *Journal of Social Work Education, 34,* 415-427.

Green, R. G. & Bentley, K. J. (1994). Attributes, experiences, and career productivity of successful social work scholars. *Social Work, 4,* 405-412.

Green, R. G. & Secret, M. (1996). Publishing by social work scholars in social work and non-social work journals. *Social Work Research, 20, 1,* 31-41.

Green, R. G. & Hayden, M. A. (2001). Citation of articles published by the most productive social work faculties in the 1990's. *Journal of Social Service Research, 27, 3,* 41-56.

Green, R. G., Baskind, F. R. & Conklin, B. (1995). The 1990s publication productivity of schools of social work with doctoral programs: "The times, are they a-changin?" *Journal of Social Work Education, 31,* 388-401.

Green, R. G. Baskind, F. R., Best, A. M. & Boyd, A. S. (1997). Getting beyond the productivity gap: Assessing variation in social work scholarship. *Journal of Social Work Education, 33,* 541-553.

Green, R. G., Baskind, F. R. & Bellin, M. H. (2002). Results of the doctoral faculty publication project: Journal article productivity and its correlates in the 1990s. *Journal of Social Work Education, 37,* 135-152.

30 BIBLIOMETRICS IN SOCIAL WORK

Green, R.G., Hutchison, E. D. & Sar, B. K. (1992). Evaluating scholarly performance: The productivity of graduates of social work doctoral programs. *Social Service Review, 66*, 441-466.

Green, R. G. Kvarfordt, C. L. & Hayden, M. A. (2001). The middle years of the Decade Publication Project: 1994-97. *Journal of Social Work Education, 35, 2*, 195-202.

Grinnell, R. M. & Royer, M. L. (1983). Authors of articles in social work journals. *Journal of Social Service Research, 3/4*, 147-154.

Holden, G., Rosenberg, G. & Barker, K. (2005). Bibliometrics: A potential decision making aid in hiring, reappointment, tenure and promotion decisions. *Social Work in Health Care*, 41(3/4), 67-92.

Hopps, J. G. (1992). A response to Pardeck: From the Past-Editor of *Social Work*. *Research on Social Work Practice, 2*, 499-500.

Howard, M. O. & Howard, D. A. (1992). Citation analysis of 541 articles published in drug and alcohol journals: 1984-1988. *Journal of Studies on Alcohol, 53*, 427-434.

Hull, G. H. & Johnson, H. W. (1994). Publication rates of undergraduate social work programs in selected journals. *Journal of Social Work Education, 30*, 34-62.

ISI (2003). *Interpretation*. Retrieved 1/13/04 from: http://esi-topics.com/interpreting.html

Jayaratne, S. (1979). Analysis of selected social work journals and productivity rankings among schools of social work. *Journal of Education for Social Work, 15, 3*, 72-80.

Johnson, H. W. & Hull, G. H. (1995). Publication productivity of BSW faculty. *Journal of Social Work Education, 31*, 358-368.

Jones, A. W. (1999). The impact of *Alcohol and Alcoholism* among substance abuse journals. *Alcohol and Alcoholism, 34, 1*, 25-34.

Jones, J. F. & Jones, L. M. (1986). Citation analysis as an approach to journal assessment in social work. *National Taiwan University Journal of Sociology, 18*, 207-219.

Karger, H. J. (1999). The politics of social work research. *Research on Social Work Practice, 9*, 96-9.

Kirk, S. A. (1984). Methodological issues in the comparative study of schools of social work. *Journal of Social Service Research, 7, 3*, 59-73.

Kirk, S. A. & Rosenblatt, A. (1980). Women's contributions to social work journals. *Social Work, May*, 204-209.

Kirk, S. A. & Rosenblatt, A. (1984). The contribution of women faculty to social work journals. *Social Work, January-February*, 67-9.

Kirk, S. A., Wasserstrum, K. & Miller, D. A. (1977). Publish and perish: A study of promotion and tenure in schools of social work. *Journal of Social Welfare, Winter*, 90-7.

Klein, W. C. & Bloom, M. (1992). Studies of scholarly productivity in social work using citation analysis. *Journal of Social Work Education, 28*, 291-299.

Kostoff, R. N. (1998). The use and misuse of citation analysis in research evaluation. *Scientometrics, 43, 1,* 27-43.

Kostoff, R. N. (2002). Citation analysis of research performer quality. *Scientometrics, 53, 1,* 49-71.

Kreuger, L. W. (1993). Should there by a moratorium on articles that rank schools of social work based on faculty publications? Yes! *Journal of Social Work Education, 29,* 240-246.

Kreuger, L. W. (1999). Shallow science? *Research on Social Work Practice, 9,* 108-110.

Kroll, H. W. (1976). Institutional sources of articles published in social work journals: 1965-1974. *Arete, 4,* 121-125.

Ligon, J. & Thyer, B. A. (2001). Academic affiliations of social work journals authors: A productivity analysis from 1994-98. *Journal of Social Service Research, 28,* 69-81.

Ligon, J., Thyer, B. A. & Dixon, D. (1995). Academic affiliations of those published in social work journals: A productivity analysis, 1989-1993. *Journal of Social Work Education, 31, 3,* 369-76.

Lindsey, D. (1976). Distinction, achievement and editorial board membership. *American Psychologist, 31,* 799-804.

Lindsey, D. (1978a). *The scientific publication system in social science.* San Francisco: Jossey-Bass.

Lindsey, D. (1978b). The corrected quality ratio: A composite index of scientific contribution to knowledge. *Social Studies of Science, 8, 3,* 349-354.

Lindsey, D. (1978c). The outlook of journal editors and referees on the normative criteria of scientific craftsmanship. *Quality and Quantity, 12,* 45-62.

Lindsey, D. (1980). Production and citation measures in the sociology of science: The problem of multiple authorship. *Social Studies of Science, 10,* 145-162.

Lindsey, D. (1982). Further evidence for adjusting for multiple authorship. *Scientometrics, 4, 5,* 389-395.

Lindsey, D. (1988). Assessing precision in the manuscript review process: A little better than a dice roll. *Scientometrics: 14, 1-2,* 75-82.

Lindsey, D. (1989). Using citation counts as a measure of quality in science: Measuring what's measurable rather than what's valid. *Scientometrics, 15,* 189-203.

Lindsey, D. (1991). Precision in the manuscript review process: Hargens and Herting revisited. *Scientometrics, 22, 2,* 313-325.

Lindsey, D. (1992). Improving the quality of social work journals: From the Editor of *Children and Youth Services Review. Research on Social Work Practice, 2,* 515-524.

Lindsey, D. (1999). Ensuring standards in social work research. *Research on Social Work Practice, 9,* 115-120.

Lindsey, D. & Kirk, S. A. (1992). The role of social work journals in the development of a knowledge base for the profession. *Social Service Review, 66,* 295-310.

*32* BIBLIOMETRICS IN SOCIAL WORK

MacRoberts, M. H. & MacRoberts, B. R. (1989). Problems of citation analysis: A critical review. *Journal of the American Society for Information Science, 40*, 342-349.

MacRoberts, M. H. & MacRoberts, B. R. (1992). Problems of citation analysis. *Social Work Research & Abstracts, 28*, 4.

MacRoberts, M. H. & MacRoberts, B. R. (1997). Citation content analysis of a botany journal. *Journal of the American Society for Information Science, 48*, 274-275.

McMurty, S. L., Rose, S. J. & Cisler, R. A. (2003). Identifying and administering the most-used rapid assessment instruments. Presentation at the Seventh Annual Society for Social Work & Research Conference, Washington, DC.

McNeece, C. A. (1981). Faculty publications, tenure, and job satisfaction in graduate social work programs. *Journal of Education for Social Work, 17, 3*, 13-19.

Meinert, R. (1993). Response to Dr. Kreuger. *Journal of Social Work Education, 29*, 245-246.

Mendelsohn, H. N. (1997). *An author's guide to social work journals.* Washington, DC: NASW Press.

Midgley, J. (1999). Academic merit, professional needs, and social work education. *Research on Social Work Practice, 9*, 104-107.

Mokau, N., Hull, G. & Burkett, S. (1993). The development of knowledge by undergraduate program directors. *Journal of Social Work Education, 29, 2*, 160-170.

Myers, C. R. (1970). Journal citations and scientific eminence in contemporary psychology. *American Psychologist, 25*, 1041-1048.

Najman, J. M. & Hewitt, B. (2003). The validity of publication and citation counts for Sociology and other selected disciplines. *Journal of Sociology, 39, 1*, 62-80.

Narin, F., Olivastro, D. & Stevens, K. A. (1994). Bibliometrics/theory, practice and problems. *Evaluation Review, 18, 1*, 65-76.

Nisonger, T. E. (2001). Report on the 8th International Conference on Scientometrics and Informetrics in Sydney, Australia. *Library Collections, Acquisitions, and Technical Services, 25*, 485-488.

Norton, M. J. (2000). *Introductory concepts in information science.* Medford, NJ: Information Today, Inc.

Oppenheim, C. (1997). The correlation between citation counts and the 1992 research assessment exercise ratings for British research in genetics, anatomy and archaeology. *Journal of Documentation, 53*, 477-487.

Pardeck, J. T., Arndt, B. J., Light, D. B., Mosley, G. F., Thomas, S. D., Werner, M. A. & Wilson, K. E. (1991). Distinction and achievement levels of editorial board members of psychology and social work journals. *Psychological Reports, 68*, 523-27.

Pardeck, J. T. (1992a). Are social work journal editorial boards competent? Some disquieting data with implications for research on social work practice. *Research on Social Work Practice, 2*, 487-96.

Pardeck, J. T. (1992b). The distinction and achievement levels of social work editorial boards revisited. *Research on Social Work Practice, 2*, 529-537.

Pardeck, J. T. (2002). Scholarly productivity of editors of social work and psychology journals. *Psychological Reports, 90*, 1051-1054.

Pardeck, J. T., Chung, W. S. & Murphy, J. W. (1995). An examination of the scholarly productivity of social work journal editorial board members and guest reviewers. *Research on Social Work Practice*, *5*, 223-234.

Pardeck, J. T. & Meinart, R. G. (1999a). Scholarly achievements of the *Social Work* editorial board and consulting editors: A commentary. *Research on Social Work Practice*, *9*, 86-91.

Pardeck, J. T. & Meinart, R. G. (1999b). Improving the scholarly quality of *Social Work's* editorial board and consulting editors: A professional obligation. *Research on Social Work Practice*, *9*, 121-127.

Phelan, T. J. (1999). A compendium of issues for citation analysis. *Scientometrics*, *45*, *1*, 117-36.

Plomp, R. (1990). The significance of the number of highly cited papers as an indicator of scientific prolificacy. *Scientometrics*, *19*, 185-197.

Porter, A. L. (1977). Citation analysis: Queries and caveats. *Social Studies of Science*, *7*, 257-67.

Rao, I. K. R. (1998). Informetrics: Scope, definition, methodology and conceptual questions. Workshop on *Informetrics and Scientometrics*, 16-19 March 1998, Bangalore. Retrieved 8/2/03 from: http://drtc.isibang.ac.in/~sneha/gsdl/AA.pdf

Reamer, F. G. (1992). A response to Pardeck: From the Editor-in-Chief of the *Journal of Social Work Education*. *Research on Social Work Practice*, *2*, 501-504.

Reamer, F. G. (1999). Social work scholarship and gatekeeping: Reflection on the debate. *Research on Social Work Practice*, *9*, 92-95.

Rehr, H., Rosenberg, G., Showers, N. & Blumenfield, S. (1998). Social work in health care: Do practitioners's writings suggest an applied social science? *Social Work in Health Care*, *28*, *2*, 63-81.

Rehr, H., Showers, N., Rosenberg, G. & Blumenfield, S. (1998). Profiles of published social work practitioners: Who wrote and why. *Social Work in Health Care*, *28*, *2*, 83-94.

Robbins, S. P., Corcoran, K. J., Hepler, S. E. & Magner, G. W. (1985). *Academic productivity in social work education*. Washington, DC: Council on Social Work Education.

Rosen, A. (1979). Evaluating doctoral programs in social work: A case study. *Social Work Research & Abstracts*, *15*, *2*, 19-27.

Rosenberg, G., Holden, G. & Barker, K (2005). What happens to our ideas? A bibliometric analysis of articles in *Social Work in Health Care* in the 1990s. *Social Work in Health Care*, 41 (3/4), 37-68.

Rothman, J., Kirk, S. A. & Knapp, H. (2003). Reputation and publication productivity among social work researchers. *Social Work Research*, *27*, 105-115.

Rousseau, R. (1997). Sitations: An exploratory study. *Cybermetrics: International Journal of Scientometrics, Informetrics and Bibliometrics*, *1*, *1*. http://www.cindoc.csic.es/cybermetrics/

Rubin, A. & Powell, D. M. (1987). Gender and publication rates: A reassessment with population data. *Social Work*, *32*, 317-320.

Saha, S., Saint, S. & Christakis, D. A. (2003). Impact factor: A valid measure of journal quality? *Journal of the Medical Library Association, 91*, 42-46.

Seaberg, J. R. (1998). Faculty reports of workload: Results of a national survey. *Journal of Social Work Education, 34*, 7-19.

Sellin, M. K. (1993). *Bibliometrics: An annotated bibliography, 1970-1990.* New York: G. K. Hall & Co.

Schiele, J. (1991). Publication productivity of African-American social work faculty. *Journal of Social Work Education, 27, 2*, 125-134.

Schoepflin, U. & Glanzel, W. (2001). Two decades of "Scientometrics": An interdisciplinary field represented by its leading journal. *Scientometrics, 50*, 301-312.

Schuerman, J. R. (1992). A response to Pardeck: From the Editor of the *Social Service Review. Research on Social Work Practice, 2*, 499-500.

Smith, S. L., Baker, D. R., Campbell, M. E. & Cunningham, M. E. (1985). An exploration of the factors shaping the scholarly productivity of social work academicians. *Journal of Social Service Research, 8, 3*, 81-99.

Staudt, M. M., Dulmus, C. & Bennett, G. A. (2003). Facilitating writing by practitioners: Survey of practitioners who have published. *Social Work, 48, 1*, 75-83.

Tague-Sutcliffe, J. (1992). An introduction to informetrics. *Information Processing & Management, 28, 1*, 1-3.

Thyer, B. A. & Bentley, K. (1986). Academic affiliations of social work authors: A citation analysis of six major journals. *Journal of Social Work Education, 22*, 67-73.

Thyer, B. A., Boynton, K. E., Bennis, L. & Levine, D. L. (1994). Academic affiliations of social work journal article authors: A publication productivity analysis from 1984-1988. *Journal of Social Service Research, 18, 3/4*, 153-167.

Thyer, B. A. & Myers, L. L. (2003). An empirical evaluation of the editorial practices of social work journals. *Journal of Social Work Education, 39, 1*, 125-140.

Thyer, B. A. & Polk, G. (1997). Social work and psychology professors' scholarly productivity: A controlled comparison of cited journal articles. *Journal of Applied Social Sciences, 21, 2*, 105-110.

Twining, J. (2002). Bibliometrics: An overview. Retrieved 11/10/02 from: *http://www.du.edu/~jtwining/LIS4326/bibliometrics.htm*

vonUngern-Sternberg, S. (2000). Scientific communication and bibliometrics. Retrieved 11/14/02 from: *http://www.abo.fi/~sungern/comm00.htm*

Williams, J. W. (2001). Journals of the century. *The Serials Librarian, 39, 3*, 69-77.

Wormell, I. (2000a). Bibliometric analysis of the welfare topic. *Scientometrics, 48*, 203-236.

Wormell, I. (2000b). Critical aspects of the Danish Welfare State–as revealed by issue tracking. *Scientometrics, 48*, 237-250.

Wouters, P. (2000). Garfield as alchemist. In B. Cronin & H. B. Atkins (Eds.), *The Web of Knowledge: A Festchrift in Honor of Eugene Garfield.* (pp. 65-72). Medford, NY: Information Today.

# What Happens to Our Ideas?
# A Bibliometric Analysis of Articles
# in *Social Work in Health Care*
# in the 1990s

Gary Rosenberg, PhD
Gary Holden, DSW
Kathleen Barker, PhD

**SUMMARY.** Scholars spend a considerable amount of time reflecting upon their professional work. When individuals decide to communicate their professional thoughts beyond informal venues, the penultimate expression of their reflection is the peer reviewed journal article. The study reported here entailed a bibliometric analysis of articles appearing in the journal *Social Work in Health*

---

Gary Rosenberg is Edith J. Baerwald Professor of Community and Preventive Medicine, Mount Sinai School of Medicine. Gary Holden is Professor, New York University. Kathleen Barker is Professor of Psychology, The City University of New York: Medgar Evers College.

Address correspondence to: Gary Rosenberg, Box 1252, Mount Sinai School of Medicine, 1 Gustave L. Levy Place, New York, NY 10029.

[Haworth co-indexing entry note]: "What Happens to Our Ideas? A Bibliometric Analysis of Articles in *Social Work in Health Care* in the 1990s." Rosenberg, Gary, Gary Holden, and Kathleen Barker. Co-published simultaneously in *Social Work in Health Care* (The Haworth Social Work Practice Press, an imprint of The Haworth Press, Inc.) Vol. 41, No. 3/4, 2005, pp. 35-66; and: *Bibliometrics in Social Work* (ed: Gary Holden, Gary Rosenberg, and Kathleen Barker) The Haworth Social Work Practice Press, an imprint of The Haworth Press, Inc., 2005, pp. 35-66. Single or multiple copies of this article are available for a fee from The Haworth Document Delivery Service [1-800-HAWORTH, 9:00 a.m. - 5:00 p.m. (EST). E-mail address: docdelivery@haworthpress.com].

Available online at http://www.haworthpress.com/web/SWHC
© 2005 by The Haworth Press, Inc. All rights reserved.
doi:10.1300/J010v41n03_02

*Care* during the 1990s, in order to better understand what happens to our ideas after they appear in a peer reviewed journal article. *[Article copies available for a fee from The Haworth Document Delivery Service: 1-800-HAWORTH. E-mail address: <docdelivery@haworthpress.com> Website: <http://www.HaworthPress.com> © 2005 by The Haworth Press, Inc. All rights reserved.]*

**KEYWORDS.** Social work in health care, journal, scholarship, bibliometrics informetrics, scientometrics, citation analysis, sociology of science, social work journals

## *INTRODUCTION*

Scholars, whether they are practitioners or academics or both, spend a substantial amount of time thinking about their professional concerns. Sometimes those thoughts are simply reflected upon, never to enter an informal or formal exchange of ideas. Other times, these thoughts are discussed with students or colleagues, and sometimes they are more formally expressed at a local, national or international professional conference. Alternatively, a scholar may express her or his ideas in a newsletter, monograph or book. Sometimes after much thought, discussion and interaction with peer reviewers, editors and copy editors, a scholar's thoughts see the light of day in a peer reviewed journal article. Yet, the publication of an article in a journal is not the end point in the life of the article.

In the social work profession, the examination of the life of articles beyond the point of publication has a history dating back at least to the 1970s (e.g., Jayaratne, 1979; Lindsey, 1976; 1978a; 1978b; Rosen, 1979). These studies used various bibliometric techniques, an approach to the study of scholarly communication that includes citation analysis. These researchers found, in part, that social work professionals tended to publish comparatively less than scholars in some other fields. Furthermore, it was also observed that the distribution of published works was positively skewed, that is, a small proportion of authors published many articles. These and other authors replicated and extended this work during the subsequent decades, with similar results. For instance, they found similar positive skewing of publication rates; that social work editorial board members did not publish very much when compared to peers in other social science professions; that individual social work academics and individual schools had quite variable rates of publication; that while social work faculty articles do get cited, they get cited less than articles by psychology faculty; and that social work faculty articles in non social work journal articles were more frequently cited than their articles in social work journals (e.g., Baker & Wilson, 1992; Fox & Faver, 1985; Green & Bentley, 1994; Green & Hayden, 2001; Green, Baskind & Bellin, 2002; Ligon & Thyer, 2001; Pardeck, Chung & Murphy, 1995; Pardeck, 2002; Robbins, Corcoran, Hepler & Magner, 1985; Thyer & Polk; 1997).

Bibliometrics have also been used to examine: libraries' social work holdings; the publication of books and dissertations in social work over time; the body of work of individuals; publications in particular content areas such as substance use and welfare; the interaction of social work and other fields; the relationships among journals in the social work journal network; the use of social science literature in social work journals; the impact of social work journals; and the relationship of citations to reputation as a social work researcher (e.g., Baker, 1991; 1992; Cheung, 1990; Bush, Epstein & Sainz, 1997; Holden, Rosenberg & Barker, 2005a; Howard & Howard, 1992; Jones & Jones, 1986; Rothman, Kirk & Knapp, 2003; Wormell, 2000a; 2000b). Key literature related to the current study will be summarized below. A comprehensive review of bibliometrics is available elsewhere (Holden, Rosenberg & Barker, 2005b).

## *Impact of Journals*

While the authors fully understand that impact can take many forms, in the current study it has been narrowly conceptualized as the impact of articles, operationalized as citations (c.f., Narin, Olivastro & Stevens, 1994). That is, the number of articles that cite the target article. Criticisms of this approach will be considered in the Discussion section.

One can examine impact using journals as the unit of analysis. One social work study (Bush, Epstein & Sainz, 1997) examined the impact of social science sources (journals and books) on three key social work journals for the 1956 to 1992 period. They found a general increase (although a decline in the last two years studied) in the number of references in the articles in these journals. The greatest mean number of references across time were to social science books, followed by social science journals.

Studies of journal impact often use the impact factor score (IFS), which is an indicator of a journal's impact that is derived from citations (Garfield, 1999). The IFS for journal X for 2002 is computed by dividing the number of citations during 2002 (in journals in the Institute for Scientific Information (ISI) Web of Science (WoS) databases) to articles in the journal X in 2000 and 2001, by the number of articles in the journal X in 2000-01 (ISI, 1994). Lindsey and Kirk (1992) examined core social work journals' IFSs and found that *Social Work* (SW) had the highest IFS during the 1981-89 period (mean = .70). To provide a more current comparison, the authors examined the IFSs for both SW and *Social Work in Health Care* (*SWHC*) from 1990-1999. SW had a mean IFS of .935 for the period and *SWHC* had a mean IFS of .276. As Lindsey and Kirk point out, such findings may be due in part to the vast differentials in the distribution of SW, relative to specialty journals. NASW (1997) reported a circulation of 163,000+ for SW and 1,007 for *SWHC*. SW had an IFS 3.4 times larger than *SWHC* during the 1990s and a reported (1997) circulation that was 161 times larger. Lindsey and Kirk's point received support from Howard and Howard (1992), who found a correlation of $r = .68$ between the journal citation rates and the size of the journals' circulation in their study of 12 substance abuse journals. Obviously, one needs to be cautious about any bibliometric indicator's psychometric properties. IFSs have received support as an indicator of journal quality (Christenson & Sigelman, 1985; Saha, Saint & Christakis, 2003), although they have been critiqued as an inappropriate indicator of an individual scholar's impact as well as for other reasons (e.g., Frank, 2003; Furr, 1995; Garfield, 1996; Glanzel & Moed, 2002).

## Impact of Journals/Articles

One can move beyond journals as the sole unit of analysis, by adding a specific focus on the articles within those journals. The Howard and Howard (1992) study mentioned above focused on 541 articles published in 12 drug and alcohol journals during 1984. They examined citations to those articles during the 1984-1988 period and found that 71.2% of the articles were cited at least once and that the mean number of citations for the group of articles was 3.48. The top five articles were cited a total of 58, 41, 39, 29 and 28 times respectively. Nieminen and Isohanni (1997) created a sample of articles from the 1987-92 period focusing on therapeutic communities, but then included analyses at the level of journals. In terms of, citations at the article level (recorded in 11/94), they reported that 39% of the articles were not cited during the study period.

Dumas, Logan and Finley's (1993) bibliometric analysis included articles from the journals *British Journal of Social Work* (BJSW) and SW during the 1984-91 period. They reported that BJSW was cited 435 times and SW was cited 2276 times during those eight years. In terms of individual articles the top five articles in BJSW were cited 16, 13, 11, 8 and 8 times respectively, whereas the top six in SW were cited 29, 27, 23, 22 and 21 (two articles) times respectively. The authors noted that using the total number of cites without controlling for time made interpretation of this finding problematic, in that for both journals, all of the highly cited articles came from the 1984-1986 period (the first three years of the study period). Other factors such as international differences in citation norms might have contributed to this finding as well.

In summary, there is a history of bibliometric research in social work that has begun to reveal the patterns of publications by individuals and the impact that scholarship has produced. These bibliometric techniques have also been used from different perspectives to increase our understanding of other aspects of scholarly communications in social work. One particular aspect that has received attention is the impact of journals and the articles within those journals. Given this intriguing prior work, it was decided to further explore what happens to our ideas through a bibliometric analyses of articles appearing in the journal *SWHC* during the 1990s. The goals were to describe the set of articles, to describe the overall impact of the set and to isolate and describe the subset of articles with the greatest impact.

## *METHOD*

### *Sample*

The sample for this study consists of articles published in the *SWHC* during the 1990-1999 period. This sample is further restricted to full length articles, including review articles (e.g., book reviews, editorials, meeting abstracts, corrections, letters, and notes were excluded). All articles in *SWHC* during this time period are covered in the Web of Science (WoS, *http://isi2.isiknowledge.com/portal.cgi/WoS*), which is the source of much of the data for this study. The WoS is a database available from Thomson's Institute for Scientific Information (*http://isi4.isiknowledge.com/portal.cgi*). In January, 2004, the WoS database covered approximately 8500 journals.

### *Time Frame*

The focus of the current study was on citations in the WoS during the 1990-2002 period, to *SWHC* articles from the 1990-1999 period. The three additional years for the citation period allows a beginning view of the impact of publications from the end of the publication period and a longer time frame in which to consider the impact of publications from earlier in the publication period. Given the amount of time that typically passes between acceptance for publication and actual publication, this approach should provide a fuller picture of an article's impact.

## Procedure

A series of General Searches were performed on the WoS for articles in *SWHC* for the period. In instances where data elements could not be coded from the WoS, clarification was sought from the original article, WWW searches (e.g., for an author's CV), and/or from *SWHC* editorial staff. Using the General Search feature allows the possibility of missing citations that have incorrect information regarding the cited article (e.g., incorrect publication years, volumes, pages numbers, etc.). Such mistakes may be discovered by using the WoS Cited Reference search. This was not done here as it would have required inferences beyond the knowledge of the authors of the current study and the authors assumed that any General Search related errors would likely be random across this population. Data from the WoS searches were then entered in to SPSS 11.0.1 for further analyses.

## Measures

The length of the article, number of authors, and number of references in the reference list of the article were recorded from the WoS search results. Additional data was obtained from the WoS search results and calculated as follows. Age of the article was operationalized as the result of subtracting the year of publication from 2002 and adding .5. The .5 was added in order to make the age estimate more accurate. Citations counts for each article were adjusted for time by dividing the citation totals by the age of the article. Two measures, lag time and persistence, were used from Klein and Bloom's (1992) work. Lag time refers to the number of years between publication and first citation (for those articles that were cited in the period under study). As with age, .5 was added to the difference to make it a better estimate of the actual lag time (see Holden, Rosenberg & Barker, 2005a for further explanation regarding this statistic). Persistence was calculated by summing the number of years in which an author's work has been cited. Persistence is obviously more difficult to interpret for more recent articles.

Six citation statistics were included in the current study: cited by self and/or co-authors on original article (c.f., Aksnes, 2003; Fortune, 1992); cited by others; and total cites. Each of these three statistics was also adjusted for the age of the publication. Diachronous self-citations (Aksnes, 2003)–instances where the article being examined was cited by the author in one of her subsequent articles–are the focus here. Because the unit of analysis is the article in this study, diachronous self-citations are those citations of the article being examined by any of the authors on that article. Synchronous self-citations are those self-citations contained in the reference list of the article being examined (Aksnes, 2003). While some self/co-author citation may be inappropriate, other instances may be scientifically appropriate (e.g., publications in a long term research program). This position is common in the bibliometric literature (e.g., Klein & Bloom, 1992). Although the analyses in the current study do not distinguish between the inappropriate and the appropriate, these analyses do provide an estimate of the overall size of this factor. The adjustment for age makes the outcomes for articles later in the time period somewhat more comparable with outcomes for articles earlier in the time period. A second time adjusted analysis will be provided. Statistics representing *concentration* (the percentage of papers that receive 50% of the citations), *citedness* (the number of citations an article needs to be in the top 1% of papers), and *uncitedness* (percentage of papers that had not been cited in the study period) were computed as well (ISI, 1999; Katz, 1999).

Dumas, Logan and Finley (1993) examined the subjects of the articles using the *Social Work Research and Abstracts* codes. That approach was considered and then discarded in the current study because of potential coding and analytic difficulties (e.g., reliability and validity). Given that the unit of analysis here is the article, adjustments for the number of authors were not used.

## *RESULTS*

### *Description of Sample*

Examination of the journal and searches of the WoS resulted in a sample of 366 articles for analysis. A series of exploratory analyses were undertaken. The number of publications per year ($M = 36.6$) was variable over the time period ranging from 21 articles in 1994 to 53 articles in both 1995 and 1997. For the entire sample, there were a total of 1291 citations to these articles during the 1990-2002 period. The overall diachronous self/co-author citation rate was 9.2% (119/1289–reduced n from missing data).

Although means are also reported in Table 1, the focus will be on medians in the text regarding Table 1, given the non-normal distributions of these variables. As can be seen, the typical article was: 16 pages long; had 2 authors; 27 references and was cited for the first time 3.5 years after publication. This typical article was cited in 2 different years after it was published and a total of 2 times. In regards to the self/co-author citation issue, the typical article was not cited in this fashion ($M = .33$; $Mdn = 0$). In terms of time adjusted impact, it can be seen that the typical article was cited .29 times per year (.27 times per year by others). How was the impact distributed across the sample of articles? It was observed that 15.8% of the papers received 50% of the citations (concentration), papers needed 20 or more citations to be in the top 1% of papers (citedness), and 20.2% of the papers had not been cited as of the end of 2002 (uncitedness).

Did the articles' structural variables, such as article length, have any relationship to the articles' impact? The number of references (*Kendall's Tau b* = .16; $r = .26$) and the number of pages (*Kendall's Tau b* = .15; $r = .26$) were significantly correlated ($p < .01$, two tailed) with the total number of citations per year.

Adair and Vohra (2003) recently reported relatively consistent increases in the number of references in articles from selected journals in psychology, sociology, biology and physics for the 1972-2000 period. The average increase across the seven journals they studied was from 39 references per article during the 1990-1992 period to 48.1 references per article during 1996-1998. The comparable mean numbers of references for *SWHC* were 27.7 and 32.7 per article during the 1990-1992 and the 1996-1998 periods, respectively (a statistically significant increase, Mann-Whitney U Test, $p < .05$).

Increases in multiple authorship of articles in social work have been noted for earlier time periods (Kirk & Rosenblatt, 1980: 1934-1977 period; Grinnell & Royer, 1983: initial publication through 1/1/79). More recently, Gelman and Gibelman (1999) reported an increase in multiple authorship between the 1973-77 and 1993-97 periods (c.f., Rubin & Chang, 2003 re: increases in multiple authorship in health economics). For *SWHC*, there was a significant increase in the number of authors per

## BIBLIOMETRICS IN SOCIAL WORK

TABLE 1. Descriptive statistics for *Social Work in Health Care* articles for 1990-1999 (n = 366).

| | N of pages | N of authors | N of references | Lag time to first citation[1] | Persistence | Self-Co-author cites | Other cites | Total cites | Self-Co-author cites per yr. | Other cites per yr. | Total cites per yr. |
|---|---|---|---|---|---|---|---|---|---|---|---|
| Minimum | 6.0 | 1 | 0 | .5 | 0 | 0 | 0 | 0 | 0 | 0 | 0 |
| Maximum | 45.0 | 9 | 163 | 11.5 | 10 | 9 | 33 | 41 | 1.38 | 2.9 | 3.6 |
| Mean (SD) | 16.8 (5.23) | 2.2 (1.48) | 31.0 (19.5) | 3.7 (1.84) | 2.3 (2.1) | .33 (.95) | 3.2 (3.97) | 3.5 (4.28) | .05 (.13) | .40 (.43) | .44 (.47) |
| Median | 16.0 | 2.0 | 27.0 | 3.5 | 2.0 | 0 | 2.0 | 2.0 | 0 | .27 | .29 |

Note. n's for some analyses are slightly smaller due to missing data for particular variables.
[1] Only articles that were cited are included in this statistic.

article between the 1990-91 time frame and 1998-99 ($M's$ = 2.0 and 2.43 respectively, Mann-Whitney U Test, $p < .05$).

### Description of High Impact Groups

In terms of high impact (as measured by citations) the ten articles with most impact (sometimes more than ten are reported due to ties) on each of four variables are identified in Table 2. The bolded numbers in each of the first four columns represent the group of articles with the highest impact for the 1990-2002 time period. Table 2 actually includes 20 articles. This was necessary because of ties and the fact that some articles were in the top ten on one, two or three of the four variables, but not all four. Seven articles were in the top ten on all four impact variables.

TABLE 2. Citation analysis of high impact articles in *Social Work in Health Care*.

| Total cites | Total cites by others | Age adjusted total cites | Age adjusted total cites by others | N of pages | N of references | Lag time to first cite | Persistence | Author(s) (publication year). Title. |
|---|---|---|---|---|---|---|---|---|
| 41 | 33 | 3.57 | 2.87 | 41 | 95 | 3.5 | 9 | Holden, G. (1991). The relationship of self-efficacy appraisals to subsequent health related outcomes: A meta-analysis. |
| 21 | 21 | 2.47 | 2.47 | 17 | 70 | 1.5 | 7 | Abbott, A. A. (1994). A feminist approach to substance-abuse treatment and service delivery. |
| 20 | 20 | 1.60 | 1.60 | 17 | 28 | 3.5 | 10 | Ahmed, F., McRae, J. A., & Ahmed, N. (1990). Factors associated with not receiving adequate prenatal care in an urban black population: program planning implications. |
| 19 | 18 | 2.00 | 1.89 | 44 | 163 | 2.5 | 7 | Holden, G., Rosenberg, G., Barker, K., Tuhrim, S., & Brenner, B. (1993). The recruitment of research participants: A review. |

TABLE 2 (continued)

| Total cites | Total cites by others | Age adjusted total cites | Age adjusted total cites by others | N of pages | N of references | Lag time to first cite | Persistence | Author(s) (publication year). Title. |
|---|---|---|---|---|---|---|---|---|
| **16** | **16** | 1.28 | 1.28 | 19 | 51 | 2.5 | 9 | Abramson, J. S. (1990). Enhancing patient participation–clinical strategies in the discharge planning process. |
| **16** | **16** | 1.28 | 1.28 | 23 | 54 | 3.5 | 7 | Siegel, K. (1990). Psychosocial oncology research. |
| **16** | 12 | 1.52 | 1.14 | 22 | 32 | 1.5 | 7 | Fillit, H. Howe, J. L., Fulop, G., Sachs, C., Sell, L., Siegel, P. Miller, M., & Butler, R. (1992). Studies of hospital social stays in the frail elderly and their relationship to the intensity of social-work intervention. |
| **15** | **15** | **1.76** | **1.76** | 19 | 24 | 3.5 | 6 | Galinsky, M. J. & Schopler, J. H. (1994). Negative experiences in support groups. |
| **15** | **15** | **1.58** | **1.58** | 15 | 43 | 2.5 | 7 | Bonuck, K. (1993). AIDS and families–cultural, psychosocial, and functional impacts. |

| | | | | | | | | |
|---|---|---|---|---|---|---|---|---|
| **15** | **15** | 1.30 | 1.30 | 18 | 26 | 2.5 | 7 | Black, R. (1991). Women's voices after pregnancy loss–couples patterns of communication and support. |
| **15** | **13** | **1.76** | **1.53** | 23 | 27 | 2.5 | 7 | Jones, J. (1994). Embodied meaning–menopause and the change of life. |
| 13 | **13** | 1.53 | **1.53** | 17 | 28 | 2.5 | 5 | Cornelius, D. S. (1994). Managed care and social-work–constructing a context and response. |
| 14 | **13** | 1.47 | 1.37 | 21 | 52 | 2.5 | 6 | Davisali, S. H., Chesler, M. A., & Chesney, B. K. (1993). Recognizing cancer as a family disease–worries and support reported by patients and spouses. |
| 13 | **13** | 1.37 | 1.37 | 18 | 30 | 2.5 | 6 | Ross, E. (1993). Preventing burn-out among social-workers employed in the field of AIDS/HIV. |
| 13 | **13** | 1.04 | 1.04 | 16 | 35 | 3.5 | 9 | Coulton, C. (1990). Research in patient and family decision-making regarding life sustaining and long term care. |

TABLE 2 (continued)

| Total cites | Total cites by others | Age adjusted total cites | Age adjusted total cites by others | N of pages | N of references | Lag time to first cite | Persistence | Author(s) (publication year). Title. |
|---|---|---|---|---|---|---|---|---|
| 11 | 9 | **2.44** | **2.00** | 14 | 34 | 1.5 | 4 | Miller, P. J., Hedlund, S. C., Murphy, K. A. (1998). Social work assessment at end of life: Practice guidelines for suicide and the terminally ill. |
| 13 | 4 | **2.00** | .62 | 27 | 29 | .5 | 5 | Buchanan, R. J. (1996). Medicaid eligibility policies for people with AIDS. |
| 9 | 9 | 1.38 | **1.38** | 13 | 18 | 3.5 | 4 | Herbert, M. & Levin, R. (1996). The advocacy role in hospital social work. |
| 7 | 6 | **1.56** | 1.33 | 19 | 71 | 2.5 | 3 | Bourjolly, J. N. (1998). Differences in religiousness among black and white women with breast cancer. |
| 7 | 6 | **1.56** | 1.33 | 19 | 36 | 2.5 | 3 | Corcoran, J. (1998). Consequences of adolescent pregnancy/parenting: A review of the literature. |

| | | | | | | | | |
|---|---|---|---|---|---|---|---|---|
| 7 | 4 | 1.04 | .62 | 13 | 18 | .5 | 3 | Minimum for higher impact group |
| 41 | 33 | 3.57 | 2.87 | 44 | 163 | 3.5 | 10 | Maximum for higher impact group |
| 15.5 (7.1) | 14.0(6.3) | 1.72(.57) | 1.53(.49) | 21.1(8.0) | 47.3(33.4) | 2.6(.83) | 6.4(2.0) | Mean (SD) for higher impact group |
| 15 | 13 | 1.56 | 1.38 | 19 | 34.5 | 2.5 | 7.0 | Median for higher impact group |
| 2.84[1] (2.8) | 2.56[1] (2.7) | .27[1] (.34) | .22[1] (.33) | 16.5[1] (4.9) | 30.1[1] (18.0) | 3.81 (1.87) | 2.1[1] (1.84) | Mean (SD) for rest of population |

Note. Bolded numbers for individual articles represent results that are in the top ten for that variable.
1. Comparison between the two groups was statistically significant at p < .00625, 1 tailed.

As can be seen for this higher impact group in Table 2, the median number of total citations was 15 (1.56 per year) and the median number of total citations by others was 13 (1.38 per year). In terms of other variables, the typical high impact group article was 19 pages in length, had 34.5 references, was first cited 2.5 years after it was published, and was cited in 7 different years subsequent to publication. While one would expect the higher impact group described in Table 2 to be different than the rest of the sample (because of the manner in which these two groups were formed), some might ask, are those differences statistically significant? The high impact group in Table 3 was therefore contrasted with the remainder of the sample and these differences are detailed in the last two rows of Table 2. To maintain an analysiswise alpha level of .05 for the eight contrasts, a Bonferroni adjustment was used (Cliff, 1987). This meant that each of the eight contrasts was tested at an alpha level of .00625 (Mann-Whitney U Test, two-tailed). All eight contrasts were statistically significant with the higher impact group having more citations (for each of the four approaches to measuring citations) as well as more pages and references in their articles. While the higher impact group articles had significantly shorter lag times and greater persistence, the meaning of these differences is less clear because of the impact of the age of articles on these measures.

In order to better understand the effect of time on these results, an alternative analysis of high impact articles controlling for the age of articles was conducted and the results are provided in Table 3. Only those articles from the same publication year are compared meaning that they have had similar amounts of time in which to be cited (c.f., Glanzel & Moed, 2002 re: citation windows). Impact data for the top 2 articles for each year from 1990-1999 are included. When two or more articles were tied for second place on a variable all of those articles are included. Articles that appeared previously in Table 2 have an abbreviated reference in the last column (authors and year), while new high impact articles making their first appearance in Table 3 have authors, year and title information in the last column. As can be seen, 15 new high impact articles appear on this list, the bulk of those being published in 1997 or

TABLE 3. Citataion analysis of high impact articles in *Social Work in Health Care* by year of publication.

| Total cites | Total cites by others | Age adjusted total cites | Age adjusted total cites by others | N of pages | N of references | Lag time to first cite | Persistence | Author(s) (publication year). Title (for entries not in Table 2). |
|---|---|---|---|---|---|---|---|---|
| **1990** | | | | | | | | |
| 20 | 20 | 1.60 | 1.60 | 17 | 28 | 3.5 | 10 | Ahmed, F., McRae, J. A., & Ahmed, N. (1990). |
| 16 | 16 | 1.28 | 1.28 | 19 | 51 | 2.5 | 9 | Abramson, J. S. (1990). |
| 16 | 16 | 1.28 | 1.28 | 23 | 54 | 3.5 | 7 | Siegel, K. (1990). |
| **1991** | | | | | | | | |
| 41 | 33 | 3.57 | 2.87 | 41 | 95 | 3.5 | 9 | Holden, G. (1991). |
| 15 | 15 | 1.30 | 1.30 | 18 | 26 | 2.5 | 7 | Black, R. (1991). |
| **1992** | | | | | | | | |
| 16 | 12 | 1.52 | 1.14 | 22 | 32 | 1.5 | 7 | Fillit, H. Howe, J. L., Fulop, G., Sachs, C., Sell, L., Siegel, P. Miller, M., & Butler, R. (1992). |
| 12 | 8 | 1.14 | .76 | 26 | 51 | 3.5 | 7 | Soskolne, V. & Auslander, G. K. (1992). Follow-up evaluation of discharge planning by social workers in an acute-care medical center in Israel. |
| 11 | 11 | 1.05 | 1.05 | 17 | 13 | 3.5 | 6 | Berkman, B., Walker, S., Bonander, E., & Holmes, W. (1992). Early unplanned readmissions to social work of elderly patients: Factors predicting who needs follow-up services. |

TABLE 3 (continued)

| Total cites | Total cites by others | Age adjusted total cites | Age adjusted total cites by others | N of pages | N of references | Lag time to first cite | Persistence | Author(s) (publication year). Title (for entries not in Table 2). |
|---|---|---|---|---|---|---|---|---|
| 11 | 11 | 1.05 | 1.05 | 22 | 23 | 2.5 | 6 | Kugelman, W. (1992). Social-work ethics in the practice arena: A qualitative study. |
| **1993** | | | | | | | | |
| 19 | 18 | 2.00 | 1.89 | 44 | 163 | 2.5 | 7 | Holden, G., Rosenberg, G., Barker, K., Tuhrim, S., & Brenner, B. (1993). |
| 15 | 15 | 1.58 | 1.58 | 15 | 43 | 2.5 | 7 | Bonuck, K. (1993). |
| **1994** | | | | | | | | |
| 21 | 21 | 2.47 | 2.47 | 17 | 70 | 1.5 | 7 | Abbott, A. A. (1994). |
| 15 | 15 | 1.76 | 1.76 | 19 | 24 | 3.5 | 6 | Galinsky, M. J. & Schopler, J. H. (1994). |
| 15 | 13 | 1.76 | 1.53 | 23 | 27 | 2.2 | 7 | Jones, J. (1994). |
| **1995** | | | | | | | | |
| 10 | 10 | 1.33 | 1.33 | 17 | 22 | 2.5 | 5 | Cushman, L. F., Evans, P. & Namerow, P. B. (1995). Occupational stress among AIDS social-service providers. |
| 10 | 10 | 1.33 | 1.33 | 16 | 31 | 3.5 | 5 | Davidson, K. W. & Foster, Z. (1995). Social work with dying and bereaved clients–helping the workers. |
| 10 | 10 | 1.33 | 1.33 | 16 | 24 | 3.5 | 4 | Frazier, P. A., Davis-Ali, S. H., & Dahl, K. E. (1995). Stressors, social support, and adjustment in kidney-transplant patients and their spouses. |

| 1996 | | | | | | | | |
|---|---|---|---|---|---|---|---|---|
| 13 | 4 | 2.00 | .62 | 27 | 29 | .5 | 5 | Buchanan, R. J. (1996). |
| 9 | 9 | 1.38 | 1.38 | 13 | 18 | 3.5 | 4 | Herbert, M. & Levin, R. (1996). |
| 7 | 7 | 1.08 | 1.08 | 17 | 19 | 4.5 | 3 | Volland, P. (1996). Social work practice in health care: Looking to the future with a different lens. |
| **1997** | | | | | | | | |
| 7 | 7 | 1.27 | 1.27 | 14 | 4 | 3.5 | 3 | Deegan, P. E. (1997). Recovery and empowerment for people with psychiatric disabilities. |
| 6 | 4 | 1.09 | .73 | 18 | 23 | 2.5 | 4 | Sormanti, M., Kayser, K., Strainchamps, E. (1997). A relational perspective of women coping with cancer: A preliminary study. |
| 5 | 5 | .91 | .91 | 8 | 18 | 1.5 | 4 | Katz, D. A. (1997). The profile of HIV infection in women: A challenge to the profession. |

## TABLE 3 (continued)

| Total cites | Total cites by others | Age adjusted total cites | Age adjusted total cites by others | N of pages | N of references | Lag time to first cite | Persistence | Author(s) (publication year). Title (for entries not in Table 2). |
|---|---|---|---|---|---|---|---|---|
| **1998** | | | | | | | | |
| 11 | 9 | 2.44 | 2.00 | 14 | 34 | 1.5 | 4 | Miller, P. J., Hedlund, S. C., Murphy, K. A. (1998). |
| 7 | 6 | 1.56 | 1.33 | 19 | 71 | 2.5 | 3 | Bourjolly, J. N. (1998). |
| 7 | 6 | 1.56 | 1.33 | 19 | 36 | 2.5 | 3 | Corcoran, J. (1998). |
| 6 | 6 | 1.33 | 1.33 | 11 | 21 | .5 | 3 | Gilbar, O. (1998). The relationship between burnout and sense of coherence in health social workers. |
| 6 | 6 | 1.33 | 1.33 | 22 | 29 | 2.5 | 3 | Furr L. A. (1998). Psycho-social aspects of serious renal disease: A review of the literature. |
| **1999** | | | | | | | | |
| 4 | 2 | 1.14 | .57 | 18 | 54 | 2.5 | 2 | Globerman, J. (1999). Hospital restructuring: Positioning social work to manage change. |
| 3 | 3 | .86 | .86 | 13 | 22 | 2.5 | 2 | Dolgin, M. J., Somer, E., Buchvald, E. & Zaizov, R. (1999). Quality of life in adult survivors of childhood cancer. |
| 3 | 3 | .86 | .86 | 20 | 61 | 1.5 | 2 | Van Hook, M. P. (1999). Women's help-seeking patterns for depression. |

later. Four articles that were included in Table 3, did not make the cut offs for inclusion in Table 3.

## DISCUSSION

This study examined a decade's worth of publications in the journal *Social Work in Health Care*. It provided descriptive data regarding these 366 articles and the 1291 citations that they received. A group of high impact articles was identified, described and compared to the remainder of the sample of articles. A second group of high impact articles for each year of publication was also described.

In the current study, fewer references per article in *SWHC* were observed compared to the mean number of references for the psychology, sociology, biology and physics journals examined by Adair and Vohra (2003). Yet, similar to Adair and Vohra (2003), the number of references per article in *SWHC* increased between the 1990-92 and 1996-98 periods. Whether this change is due to the expansion of the body of information in the social sciences, the ease of electronic retrieval, other changes in scholar's referencing practices, some combination of these, or perhaps other factors that can not be determined from the data collected in the current study, remains to be determined. The observation in the current study that the population of articles had fewer references than other fields is consistent with Lindsey's (1978a) early findings about social work journal articles.

A number of other authors have reported increases in multiple authorship as noted above. There was a statistically significant increase in the number of authors per article in *SWHC* between 1990-91 and 1998-99, which is consistent with prior findings. Given technology facilitated increases in regional, national and international collaboration, this is not a surprising change.

With the cautions of many bibliometricians regarding inter-field comparisons firmly in mind, we note that Howard and Howard (1992) found that 28.8% of the 1984 drug and alcohol journal articles in their

*56*                BIBLIOMETRICS IN SOCIAL WORK

study had not been cited during the study period and that the mean number of citations for the sample was 3.48. The top five articles were cited a total of 58, 41, 39, 29 and 28 times respectively. Nieminen and Isohanni (1997) reported that 39% of the therapeutic community articles they examined were not cited during the study period. Dumas, Logan and Finley (1993) found that the top five articles in BJSW were cited 16, 13, 11, 8 and 8 times respectively, whereas the top five in SW were cited 29, 27, 23, 22 and 21 (two articles) times respectively. In the current study, 20.2% of the papers had not been cited, the mean number of citations was 3.5, and the top five papers were cited 41, 21, 20, 19 and sixteen times respectively. In addition to the cautions mentioned above, readers should remember that the time periods covered in these comparison studies (1984-1988, 1987-94 and 1984-91 respectively) were shorter than the period in the current study (1990-02).

What predicts the amount of impact that will be produced by an article? The number of references and number of pages were significantly correlated with the total number of citations received per year for this set of *SWHC* articles *(r's = .26 & .26)*. In other words, the greater the number of references, and the greater the length of an article, the more likely it was to be cited. In their study of 448 journal articles in psychiatry journals, Meittunen and Nieminen (2003) found that topic, study design, country of correspondence and number of authors were predictive of the number of citations. Perhaps other features of studies/articles that were not measured in the current study (e.g., primary research versus other; review article versus other; populations covered; etc.) would be more predictive of impact than the variables considered here. It will be important in such studies in the future to look at a set of articles with equivalent follow up periods (in which to determine impact). This area of study merits future investigation.

In terms of the subset of high impact articles, there was some change in the articles included in the top ten depending on the statistic used in Table 2. Some articles shifted position within the top ten, some dropped out and some were added depending on the analysis. Even though the adjustment for time makes the results more comparable for articles at the beginning and end of the time period, they still are not entirely comparable. This is born out in Table 3. When the analysis focuses on the top two articles from each year, 15 new articles were included in the high impact group. As alluded to above, the distribution of citations for any two articles from different years may be quite different and therefore it may be difficult to compare their relative impact until some distant point in the future when neither continues to be cited.

In terms of caveats, some readers may be thinking that the current study misses some of the impact produced by social workers' ideas. It does. Social workers' ideas have impact on the field via activities such as discussions with students and colleagues; teaching and supervision; presentations at a local, national or international conferences; publication in newsletters, monographs, books or in a variety of Internet outlets. But the mechanisms for studying the impact of such venues are less developed. More important to us is the issue of the quality of the venue used to disseminate ideas. Despite the fact that peer review for journals can be problematic (cf., Lindsey, 1978b; 1988; 1991; 1999; Pardeck & Meinart, 1999; Thyer & Myers, 2003), we would argue that it is the system that produces the highest quality results. Seipel (2003) recently examined social work academics perceptions of the relative value of different types of publication when making tenure decisions. He found that peer reviewed venues were considered more valuable and that peer reviewed journal articles were considered the most valuable overall. So not only do we have evidence that peer reviewed journal articles are considered the most valuable venue for publication, this is the venue for which we have a mechanism to study impact via bibliometrics (the WoS databases). *There may be many ways of saying what we know, but they are not all equal.*

The current study focused on only a single, peer reviewed journal, but did so for longer time periods than studies such as Howard and Howard (1992) or Dumas, Logan and Finley (1993). The limitations of bibliometric analyses have been noted elsewhere by both ourselves and others (e.g., Baker, 1990; 1991; Cnaan, Caputo & Shmuely, 1994; Holden, Rosenberg & Barker, 2005a; Kirk, 1984; Krueger, 1993; 1999; Lindsey, 1978a; 1980; 1982; 1989; MacRoberts & MacRoberts, 1989;

Phelan, 1999). A number of these potential limitations do not seem relevant to the current study.

For instance, the focus in this study was not on the quantity of publications by individuals or schools, but rather on the impact of publications in a *single* journal. The current study did not rely on authors' self reports regarding publications, but rather proceeded from the actual publication in the public record. While some critics have noted that the WoS does not contain all journals, this criticism does not apply here in that *SWHC* is covered in the WoS for the entire 1990-99 period. As noted by MacRoberts and MacRoberts (1989), homonyms (authors sharing the same last name and initials) and synonyms (e.g., different initials used by the same author) are potential problems in a study such as this, but we are confident in our coding, since in the majority of instances where there were questions, the answers could be determined by examining the original article, searching the WWW (faculty CVs are often posted now) or asking the *SWHC* editorial staff. The study was confined to one professional area–health social work–and thereby avoids/minimizes the concern that bibliometric comparisons across fields may be invalid due to different citation patterns in different fields (cf., Narin, Olivastro & Stevens, 1994).

On the other hand, both general research design and more specific bibliometrics related caveats may be relevant. While this was a sample of articles with virtually no missing data, it is a sample of a specific journal's articles from a specific time period, and therefore the results may not generalize to other journals or other time periods for this journal. In terms of concerns regarding bibliometrics, critics in the past have suggested that authors may be referencing work that is incorrect, not referencing the best work, or not correctly referencing satisfactory work. This may have occurred in relation to the articles in *SWHC* during this time period. There are no apparent reasons why this potential bias would be more or less of a factor for *SWHC* than any other journal. Second, we have seen no evidence that this bias in fact occurs in the social work literature and therefore would suggest that until such evidence has been reported, the profession act under the assumption that most authors value their reputation for quality work and know that this reputation is put on the line each time they publish. Therefore, they should be motivated to cite others work appropriately, as they are always at risk for exposure for doing otherwise (cf., Franck, 2002). A potential concern that is beyond the scope of this article is that citation analysis may not reflect the impact a journal has on professionals who are reading it (but not writing and citing it).

Lindsey (1989) has suggested that citation counts may be best at distinguishing articles at the upper and lower ends of the distribution, based on the distributions he observed in a number of fields. He states "[t]he difference between the article that attracts no citations and one that attracts two or three over a seven-year period is not that substantial. Thus, in the heavily populated middle range of the continuum of quality, citation counts are of doubtful utility" (p. 196). Cole (2000) notes that he and his colleagues have voiced similar concerns, as have others (Kostoff, 2002; Plomp, 1990). Yet, some might argue that citations are clearly discernable units on a ratio level scale that has an absolute zero point and equal intervals. These are psychometric questions worthy of further attention.

Finally, it has been previously noted that authors may be referencing themselves and thereby inflating citation rates. While the current study can not address the issue of appropriateness of self/co-author citation, it does provide a glimpse at the overall effect of this behavior. The rate of diachronous self/co-author citation rate was 9.2% for the entire sample. The number of self/co-author cites ranged from 0 to 9 (0-1.38 per year) with a mean of .33 (.05 per year). Aksnes (2003) examined a sample of over 45,000 Norwegian science publications from the 1981-1996 period and found that the diachronous self-citation (self and co-author combined) rate for the overall data set was 21% (minimum: 17%; maximum: 31%; psychology/psychiatry: 21%). Although the rate of self-citation in this sample is less than the rates found by Askness, further examination of the prevalence of this phenomena, in different journals and different time periods in social work is warranted.

The study presented here represents only one approach to using bibliometric indicators to examine at a journal's impact. For instance, Furr (1995) explored the impact of 22 well known social work journals by examining the IFS for each and comparing that to a sociological bibliometric measure–core influence (CI). CI focuses on citation to the target journal from core journals for the profession of interest. In Furr's study, self-citations from a core journal to itself were excluded. Furr used 1991 data and reported that *SWHC* had an IFS of .180 (rank of 14 in this set of journals). Yet, when Furr computed the CI measure, *SWHC*'s rank in this set of journals improved to 11. This is yet another example of the utility of bibliometric methods for summarizing large bodies of raw data into more comprehensible forms. The range of potential bibliometric research topics is quite broad.

In conclusion, scholars assume that colleagues read, think about and use their ideas. But that is often an assumption. Bibliometric analysis allows us to move a bit beyond that assumption, to better answer the question: *What happens to our ideas?*

## REFERENCES

Abbott, A. A. (1994). A feminist approach to substance-abuse treatment and service delivery. *Social Work in Health Care, 19, 3/4,* 67-83.

Abramson, J. S. (1990). Enhancing patient participation–clinical strategies in the discharge planning process. *Social Work in Health Care, 14, 4,* 53-71.

Adair, J. G. & Vohra, N. (2003). The explosion of knowledge, references, and citations: Psychology's unique response to a crisis. *American Psychologist, 58,* 15-23.

Ahmed, F., McRae, J. A. & Ahmed, N. (1990). Factors associated with not receiving adequate prenatal care in an urban black population: Program planning implications. *Social Work in Health Care, 14, 3,* 107-123.

Aksnes, D. (2003). A macro study of self-citation. *Scientometrics, 56,* 235-246.

Baker, D. R. (1990). Citation analysis: A methodological review. *Social Work Research & Abstracts, 26,* 3-10.

Baker, D. R. (1991). On-line bibliometric analysis for researchers and educators. *Journal of Social Work Education, 27,* 41-47.

Baker, D. R. (1992). A structural analysis of the social work journal network: 1985-1986. *Journal of Social Service Research, 15,* 153-168.

Baker, D. R. & Wilson, M. V. K. (1992). An evaluation of the scholarly productivity of doctoral graduates. *Journal of Social Work Education, 28,* 204-213.

Berkman, B., Walker, S., Bonander, E. & Holmes, W. (1992). Early unplanned readmissions to social work of elderly patients: Factors predicting who needs follow-up services. *Social Work in Health Care, 17, 4*, 103-119.

Black, R. (1991). Women's voices after pregnancy loss–couples patterns of communication and support. *Social Work in Health Care, 16, 2*, 107-123.

Bonuck, K. (1993). AIDS and families–cultural, psychosocial, and functional impacts. *Social Work in Health Care, 18*, 75-89.

Bourjolly, J. N. (1998). Differences in religiousness among black and white women with breast cancer. *Social Work in Health Care, 28*, 21-39.

Buchanan, R. J. (1996). Medicaid eligibility policies for people with AIDS. *Social Work in Health Care, 23, 2*, 15-41.

Bush, I., Epstein, I. & Sainz, A. (1997). The use of social science sources in social work practice journals: An application of citation analysis. *Social Work Research, 21, 1*, 45-56.

Cheung, K. M. (1990). Interdisciplinary relationships between social work and other disciplines: A citation study. *Social Work Research and Abstracts, 26, 3*, 23-9.

Christenson, J.A. & Sigelman, L. (1985). Accrediting knowledge: Journal stature and citation impact in social science. *Social Science Quarterly, 66*, 964-975.

Cliff, N. (1987). *Analyzing multivariate data.* New York: Harcourt Brace.

Cnaan, R. A., Caputo, R. K. & Shmuely, Y. (1994). Senior faculty perceptions of social work journals. *Journal of Social Work Education, 30*, 185-199.

Cole, J. R. (2000). A short history of the use of citations as a measure of the impact of scientific and scholarly work. In B. Cronin & H. B. Atkins (Eds.), *The Web of Knowledge: A Festschrift in Honor of Eugene Garfield.* (pp. 281-300). Medford, NY: Information Today.

Corcoran, J. (1998). Consequences of adolescent pregnancy/parenting: A review of the literature. *Social Work in Health Care, 27*, 49-67.

Coulton, C. (1990). Research in patient and family decision-making regarding life sustaining and long term care. *Social Work in Health Care, 15*, 63-78.

Cushman, L. F., Evans, P. & Namerow, P. B. (1995). Occupational stress among AIDS social-service providers. *Social Work in Health Care, 21, 3*, 115-131.

Davidson, K. W. & Foster, Z. (1995). Social work with dying and bereaved clients–helping the workers. *Social Work in Health Care, 21, 4*, 1-16.

Davisali, S. H., Chesler, M. A. & Chesney, B. K. (1993). Recognizing cancer as a family disease–worries and support reported by patients and spouses. *Social Work in Health Care, 19*, 45-65.

Deegan, P. E. (1997). Recovery and empowerment for people with psychiatric disabilities. *Social Work in Health Care, 25, 3*, 11-24.

Dolgin, M. J., Somer, E., Buchvald, E. & Zaizov, R. (1999). Quality of life in adult survivors of childhood cancer. *Social Work in Health Care, 28, 4*, 31-43.

Dumas, T., Logan, E. & Finley, A. (1993). In focus: Using citation analysis and subject classification to identify and monitor trends within a discipline. In S. Bonzi (Ed.),

*Proceedings of the 56th Annual Meeting of the American Society for Information Science.* (pp. 135-50). Medford, NJ: Learned Information, Inc.

Fillit, H., Howe, J. L., Fulop, G., Sachs, C., Sell, L., Siegel, P., Miller, M. & Butler, R. (1992). Studies of hospital stays in the frail elderly and their relationship to the intensity of social-work intervention. *Social Work in Health Care, 18, 1,* 1-22.

Fortune, A. E. (1992). More is not better–manuscript reviewer competence and citations: From the Past Editor-in-Chief of *Journal of Social Work Education. Research on Social Work Practice, 2,* 505-510.

Fox, M. F. & Faver, C. A. (1985). Men, women, and publication productivity: Patterns among social work academics. *Sociological Quarterly, 26,* 537-549.

Franck, M. (2002). Impact factors: Arbiter of excellence. *Journal of the American Medical Library Association, 91,* 4-6.

Frank, M. (2003). Impact factors: Arbiter of excellence. *Journal of the American Medical Library Association, 91,* 4-6.

Frazier, P. A., Davis-Ali, S. H. & Dahl, K. E. (1995). Stressors, social support, and adjustment in kidney-transplant patients and their spouses. *Social Work in Health Care, 21, 2,* 93-108.

Furr, A. L. (1995). The relative influence of social work journals: Impact factors vs. core influence. *Journal of Social Work Education, 31,* 38-45.

Furr, L. A. (1998). Psycho-social aspects of serious renal disease: A review of the literature. *Social Work in Health Care, 27, 3,* 97-118.

Galinsky, M. J. & Schopler, J. H. (1994). Negative experiences in support groups. *Social Work in Health Care, 20, 1,* 77-95.

Garfield, E. (1996). How can impact factors be improved? *BMJ, 313, 7054,* 411-413.

Garfield, E. (1999). Journal impact factor: A brief review. *Canadian Medical Association Journal, 161,* 979-980.

Gelman, S. R. & Gibelman, M. (1999). A quest for citations? An analysis of and commentary on the trend toward multiple authorship. *Journal of Social Work Education, 35,* 203-213.

Gilbar, O. (1998). The relationship between burnout and sense of coherence in health social workers. *Social Work in Health Care, 26, 3,* 39-49.

Glanzel, W. & Moed, H. F. (2002). Journal impact measures in bibliometric research. *Scientometrics, 53, 2,* 171-193.

Globerman, J. (1999). Hospital restructuring: Positioning social work to manage change. *Social Work in Health Care, 28, 4,* 13-30.

Green, R. G. & Bentley, K. J. (1994). Attributes, experiences, and career productivity of successful social work scholars. *Social Work, 4,* 405-412.

Green, R. G. & Hayden, M. A. (2001). Citation of articles published by the most productive social work faculties in the 1990's. *Journal of Social Service Research, 27, 3,* 41-56.

Green, R. G., Baskind, F. R. & Bellin, M. H. (2002). Results of the doctoral faculty publication project: Journal article productivity and its correlates in the 1990s. *Journal of Social Work Education, 37,* 135-152.

Grinnell, R. M. & Royer, M. L. (1983). Authors of articles in social work journals. *Journal of Social Service Research, 3/4*, 147-154.

Herbert, M. & Levin, R. (1996). The advocacy role in hospital social work. *Social Work in Health Care, 22, 3*, 71-83.

Holden, G. (1991). The relationship of self-efficacy appraisals to subsequent health related outcomes: A meta-analysis. *Social Work in Health Care, 16*, 53-93.

Holden, G., Rosenberg, G., Barker, K., Tuhrim, S. & Brenner, B. (1993). The recruitment of research participants: A review. *Social Work in Health Care, 19*, 1-44.

Holden, G., Rosenberg, G. & Barker, K. (2005a). Tracing thought through time and space: A selective review of bibliometrics in social work. *Social Work in Health Care 41 (3/4)*, 1-35.

Holden, G., Rosenberg, G. & Barker, K. (2005b). Bibliometrics: A potential decision making aid in hiring, reappointment, tenure and promotion decisions. *Social Work in Health Care. 41(3/4)*, 69-195.

Howard, M. O. & Howard, D. A. (1992). Citation analysis of 541 articles published in drug and alcohol journals: 1984-1988. *Journal of Studies on Alcohol, 53*, 427-434.

ISI (1994). The impact factor. Retrieved 7/21/03 from: http://www.isinet.com/cgi-bin/htm_hl?DB=ISIsite&STEMMER=en&WORDS=impact+factor+&COLOUR=Purple&STYLE=s&URL=http://sunweb.isinet.com/isi/hot/essays/journalcitationreports/7.html#muscat_highlighter_first_match

ISI (1999). Citations reveal concentrated influence: Some fields have it, but what does it mean? *Science Watch, Jan-Feb*, 1-2.

Jayaratne, S. (1979). Analysis of selected social work journals and productivity rankings among schools of social work. *Journal of Education for Social Work, 15, 3*, 72-80.

Jones, J. (1994). Embodied meaning–menopause and the change of life. *Social Work in Health Care, 19*, 43-65.

Jones, J. F. & Jones, L. M. (1986). Citation analysis as an approach to journal assessment in social work. *National Taiwan University Journal of Sociology, 18*, 207-219.

Katz, D. A. (1997). The profile of HIV infection in women: A challenge to the profession. *Social Work in Health Care, 24, 3/4*, 127-134.

Katz, J. S. (1999). Bibliometric indicators and the social sciences. Retrieved 7/27/03 from: http://www.sussex.ac.uk/Users/sylvank/pubs/ESRC.pdf

Kirk, S. A. (1984). Methodological issues in the comparative study of schools of social work. *Journal of Social Service Research, 7, 3*, 59-73.

Kirk, S. A. & Rosenblatt, A. (1980). Women's contributions to social work journals. *Social Work, May*, 204-209.

Klein, W. C. & Bloom, M. (1992). Studies of scholarly productivity in social work using citation analysis. *Journal of Social Work Education, 28*, 291-299.

Kostoff, R. N. (2002). Citation analysis of research performer quality. *Scientometrics, 53, 1*, 49-71.

Kreuger, L. W. (1993). Should there by a moratorium on articles that rank schools of social work based on faculty publications? Yes! *Journal of Social Work Education, 29,* 240-246.

Kreuger, L. W. (1999). Shallow science? *Research on Social Work Practice, 9,* 108-110.

Kugelman, W. (1992). Social-work ethics in the practice arena: A qualitative study. *Social Work in Health Care, 17, 4,* 59-80.

Ligon, J. & Thyer, B. A. (2001). Academic affiliations of social work journals authors: A productivity analysis from 1994-98. *Journal of Social Service Research, 28,* 69-81.

Lindsey, D. (1976). Distinction, achievement and editorial board membership. *American Psychologist, 31,* 799-804.

Lindsey, D. (1978a). *The scientific publication system in social science.* San Francisco: Jossey-Bass.

Lindsey, D. (1978b). The outlook of journal editors and referees on the normative criteria of scientific craftsmanship. *Quality and Quantity, 12,* 45-62.

Lindsey, D. (1980). Production and citation measures in the sociology of science: The problem of multiple authorship. *Social Studies of Science, 10,* 145-162.

Lindsey, D. (1982). Further evidence for adjusting for multiple authorship. *Scientometrics, 4, 5,* 389-395.

Lindsey, D. (1988). Assessing precision in the manuscript review process: A little better than a dice roll. *Scientometrics: 14, 1-2,* 75-82.

Lindsey, D. (1989). Using citation counts as a measure of quality in science: Measuring what's measurable rather than what's valid. *Scientometrics, 15,* 189-203.

Lindsey, D. (1991). Precision in the manuscript review process: Hargens and Herting revisited. *Scientometrics, 22, 2,* 313-325.

Lindsey, D. (1999). Ensuring standards in social work research. *Research on Social Work Practice, 9,* 115-120.

Lindsey, D. & Kirk, S. A. (1992). The role of social work journals in the development of a knowledge base for the profession. *Social Service Review, 66,* 295-310.

MacRoberts, M. H. & MacRoberts, B. R. (1989). Problems of citation analysis: A critical review. *Journal of the American Society for Information Science, 40,* 342-349.

Meittunen, J. & Nieminen, P. (2003). The effect of statistical methods and study reporting characteristics on the number of citations: A study of four general psychiatric journals. *Scientometrics, 57,* 377-88.

Miller, P. J., Hedlund, S. C. & Murphy, K. A. (1998). Social work assessment at end of life: Practice guidelines for suicide and the terminally ill. *Social Work In Health Care, 26, 4,* 23-36.

Narin, F., Olivastro, D. & Stevens, K. A. (1994). Bibliometrics/theory, practice and problems. *Evaluation Review, 18, 1,* 65-76.

NASW (1997). *An author's guide to social work journals.* Washington, DC: NASW Press.

Nieminen, P. & Isohanni, M. (1997). The use of bibliometric data in evaluating research on therapeutic community for addictions and psychiatry. *Substance Use & Misuse, 32,* 555-570.

Pardeck, J. T. (2002). Scholarly productivity of editors of social work and psychology journals. *Psychological Reports, 90*, 1051-1054.

Pardeck, J. T., Chung, W. S. & Murphy, J. W. (1995). An examination of the scholarly productivity of social work journal editorial board members and guest reviewers. *Research on Social Work Practice, 5*, 223-234.

Pardeck, J. T. & Meinart, R. G. (1999). Improving the scholarly quality of *Social Work's* editorial board and consulting editors: A professional obligation. *Research on Social Work Practice, 9*, 121-127.

Phelan, T. J. (1999). A compendium of issues for citation analysis. *Scientometrics, 45, 1*, 117-36.

Plomp, R. (1990). The significance of the number of highly cited papers as an indicator of scientific prolificacy. *Scientometrics, 19*, 185-197.

Robbins, S. P., Corcoran, K. J., Hepler, S. E. & Magner, G. W. (1985). *Academic productivity in social work education*. Washington, DC: Council on Social Work Education.

Rosen, A. (1979). Evaluating doctoral programs in social work: A case study. *Social Work Research & Abstracts, 15, 4*, 19-27.

Ross, E. (1993). Preventing burnout among social-workers employed in the field of AIDS/HIV. *Social Work in Health Care, 18*, 91-108.

Rothman, J., Kirk, S. A. & Knapp, H. (2003). Reputation and publication productivity among social work researchers. *Social Work Research, 27*, 105-115.

Rubin, R. M. & Chang, C. F. (2003). A bibliometric analysis of health economics articles in the economics literature: 1991-2000. *Health Economics, 12*, 403-414.

Saha, S., Saint, S. & Christakis, D. A. (2003). Impact factor: A valid measure of journal quality? *Journal of the Medical Library Association, 91*, 42-46.

Seipel, M. M. O. (2003). Assessing publication for tenure. *Journal of Social Work Education, 39*, 79-90.

Siegel, K. (1990). Psychosocial oncology research. *Social Work in Health Care, 15, 1*, 21-43.

Sormanti, M., Kayser, K. & Strainchamps, E. (1997). A relational perspective of women coping with cancer: A preliminary study. *Social Work in Health Care, 25, 1/2*, 89-106.

Soskolne, V. & Auslander, G. K. (1992). Follow-up evaluation of discharge planning by social workers in an acute-care medical center in Israel. *Social Work in Health Care, 18, 2*, 23-48.

Thyer, B. A. & Polk, G. (1997). Social work and psychology professors' scholarly productivity: A controlled comparison of cited journal articles. *Journal of Applied Social Sciences, 21, 2*, 105-110.

Thyer, B. A. & Myers, L. L. (2003). An empirical evaluation of the editorial practices of social work journals. *Journal of Social Work Education, 39, 1*, 125-140.

Van Hook, M. P. (1999). Women's help-seeking patterns for depression. *Social Work in Health Care, 29, 1*, 15-34.

66  *BIBLIOMETRICS IN SOCIAL WORK*

Volland, P. (1996). Social work practice in health care: Looking to the future with a different lens. *Social Work in Health Care, 24, 1/2*, 35-51.

Wormell, I. (2000a). Bibliometric analysis of the welfare topic. *Scientometrics, 48*, 203-236.

Wormell, I. (2000b). Critical aspects of the Danish Welfare State–as revealed by issue tracking. *Scientometrics, 48*, 237-250.

# Bibliometrics:
# A Potential Decision Making Aid in Hiring, Reappointment, Tenure and Promotion Decisions

Gary Holden, DSW
Gary Rosenberg, PhD
Kathleen Barker, PhD

**SUMMARY.** The assessment of scholarship assumes a central role in the evaluation of individual faculty, educational programs and academic fields. Because the production and assessment of scholarship is so central to the faculty role, it is incumbent upon decision makers to strive to make assessments of scholarship fair and equitable. This paper will focus on an approach to the assessment of the quantity and impact of the most important subset of an individual's scholarship–peer-reviewed journal articles. The

---

Gary Holden is Professor, New York University. Gary Rosenberg is Edith J. Baerwald Professor of Community and Preventive Medicine, Mount Sinai School of Medicine. Kathleen Barker is Professor of Psychology, The City University of New York: Medgar Evers College.

Address correspondence to Gary Holden, DSW, Room 407, MC: 6112, New York University, School of Social Work, 1 Washington Square North, New York, NY 10003 (E-mail: gary.holden@nyu.edu.

[Haworth co-indexing entry note]: "Bibliometrics: A Potential Decision Making Aid in Hiring, Reappointment, Tenure and Promotion Decisions." Holden, Gary, Gary Rosenberg, and Kathleen Barker. Co-published simultaneously in *Social Work in Health Care* (The Haworth Social Work Practice Press, an imprint of The Haworth Press, Inc.) Vol. 41, No. 3/4, 2005, pp. 67-92; and: *Bibliometrics in Social Work* (ed: Gary Holden, Gary Rosenberg, and Kathleen Barker) The Haworth Social Work Practice Press, an imprint of The Haworth Press, Inc., 2005, pp. 67-92. Single or multiple copies of this article are available for a fee from The Haworth Document Delivery Service [1-800-HAWORTH, 9:00 a.m. - 5:00 p.m. (EST). E-mail address: docdelivery@haworthpress.com].

Available online at http://www.haworthpress.com/web/SWHC
© 2005 by The Haworth Press, Inc. All rights reserved.
doi:10.1300/J010v41n03_03

*68*　　　　*BIBLIOMETRICS IN SOCIAL WORK*

primary goal of this paper is to stimulate discussion regarding scholarship assessment in hiring, reappointment, tenure and promotion decisions. *[Article copies available for a fee from The Haworth Document Delivery Service: 1-800-HAWORTH. E-mail address: <docdelivery@haworthpress.com> Website: <http:// www.HaworthPress.com> © 2005 by The Haworth Press, Inc. All rights reserved.]*

**KEYWORDS.** Hiring, reappointment, tenure and promotion decisions, faculty, scholarship, bibliometric, informetrics, scientometrics, citation analysis, sociology of science, tenure, promotion, social work education

## *INTRODUCTION*

A substantial portion of academic life focuses on the assessment of scholarship. For instance, in their roles as editors, editorial board members, consulting editors, guest reviewers, reviewers for conference submissions, book proposal reviewers, external reviewers and grant proposal reviewers, as well as their service on hiring, reappointment, tenure and promotion committees, faculty assess the work of others. The assessment of scholarship assumes a central role in the evaluation of individual faculty, educational programs and academic fields (e.g., Baker & Wilson, 1992; Bloom & Klein, 1995; Jayaratne, 1979; Kirk, 1984; Lindsey, 1976; 1978a; Pardeck, 2002; Sansone, Bedics & Rappe, 2000; Thyer & Bentley, 1986). Scholarship has assumed an increasingly important role in promotion and tenure decisions (e.g., Gibbs & Locke, 1989; Green, 1998; Harrison, Sowers-Hoag & Postley, 1989; Marsh, 1992). Scholarship is important enough in social work to have prompted the creation of Virginia Commonwealth University's *Doctoral Faculty Decade Publication Project* which contrasts schools of social work in terms of their scholarship (e.g., Green, Baskind & Conklin, 1995; Green, Baskind, Best & Boyd, 1997; Green, Baskind & Bellin, 2002; Green & Hayden, 2001; Green, Karfordt & Hayden, 1999).

Because the production and assessment of scholarship is so central to the faculty role, it is incumbent upon decision makers to strive to make assessments of scholarship more informed, more fair. This paper focuses on a particular subset of faculty: full-time, tenured and tenure-track faculty with (or seeking) appointments in colleges and universities where scholarship is an expectation. The focal points of the paper are meaningful in instances of hiring, reappointment, tenure and promotion decisions in which individuals have amassed a body of scholarship that can be assessed (e.g., the entire approach proposed below will likely not be relevant for hiring at the Assistant Professor level).

The motivation for this review of the area originated from our collective experiences in the assessment of individuals across a variety of academic settings and situations. The level of subjectivity observed in these assessments can be distressing (c.f., Garfield, 1983a; Klein & Bloom, 1992; Lindsey, 1999; Singer, 2002). These are the most important decisions in academics' lives. They should be as free from bias as possible. But that is not what happens in untold instances. Furthermore, these concerns are not new. Kirk, Wasserstrum and Miller (1977) began their study of 76 tenure and promotion decisions in 27 schools of social work with the sense that "schools have developed refined methods of applying vague generalities" (p. 89) and found little evidence to disconfirm this notion. From what we have observed (an admittedly restricted view), little seems to have changed in the past 25 years. In our own experience, stellar candidates for tenure and promotion are rejected outright on occasion; others, with more production of spin than knowledge, easily pass at times.

How can we move beyond this situation? Obviously, these decisions about potential and current full-time colleagues involve more than an assessment of their scholarship. Typically, these assessments involve teaching and service as well. But, poor instructors should be eliminated prior to tenure decisions, and service has typically had a tertiary role in this triumvirate of factors. While decisions regarding teaching and service are important, they are beyond the scope of this paper.

Seipel (2003) commented that:

70 *BIBLIOMETRICS IN SOCIAL WORK*

Because standards and expectations for tenure vary from school to school, a universal and objective standard is not feasible. However, an assessment of the values placed on the publication record of tenure candidates can prove helpful to everyone who is involved in the process. . . . All publications are not alike, and therefore each should be evaluated according to its merits. (p. 87)

Not only are all publications not alike (e.g., journal articles vs. books), there is variation within types of publication. This paper will focus on assessment of the quantity and impact of what many would argue is the most important subset of an individual's scholarship–peer reviewed journal articles (e.g., Kirk, 1991; Kostoff, 1996). This claim of primary importance of journal articles was most recently supported by the results of Seipel's (2003) survey of full-time social work faculty.

## *BIBLIOMETRICS*

The idea of more quantified evaluations of faculty seeking promotion has existed for some time (e.g., Garfield, 1983a; 1983b). How can this idea be enacted? Bibliometrics are research techniques that are used across a wide variety of fields to study publications and their byproducts (Baker, 1991; Norton, 2000; Sellen, 1993; Twining, 2002). A detailed review of bibliometrics and their use in social work have been presented in this issue, along with a new example of their use (Holden, Rosenberg & Barker, 2005; Rosenberg, Holden & Barker, 2005). *Citation analysis* is a bibliometric technique that involves assessment of the connections between publications. There have been indications over time that citations of an individual's scholarship are important in the assessment of social work and non-social work (e.g., Hargens & Schuman, 1990) faculty. For instance, the social work deans surveyed in Euster and Weinbach's (1986) study reported that citations were the 4th most important out of 15 factors in assessing the quality of journal publications (behind whether or not the journal was (1) peer reviewed or (2) major; and whether or not the article was (3) full length). A related finding from this series of studies (Euster & Weinbach, 1983; 1994) was that while publication was ranked as the second most important faculty activity in their 1981 survey (behind teaching), it was ranked as most important in the 1992 survey. While citation analysis has primarily been used within social work to examine the quantity and the impact of the work of individuals and academic institutions, some have employed the technique to answer other research questions regarding scholarship related to social work (e.g., Baker, 1991; 1992; Bush, Epstein & Sainz, 1997; Cheung, 1990; Howard & Howard, 1992; Jones & Jones, 1986; McMurty, Rose & Cisler, 2003; Rothman, Kirk & Knapp, 2003; Wormell, 2000a; 2000b).

In one of the most direct forerunners of the work reported here, Klein and Bloom (1992) also sought to help the profession reduce the level of subjectivity in tenure and promotion decisions. They reported four studies using citation analysis. In the first study of social work experts (authors in the *Encyclopedia of Social Work*), they found that in 1987, on average, these experts were cited 9.4 times per person. Among academics, full professors (13.7) were cited more than associate professors (7.6) and assistant professors (4.7). In their second study, Klein and Bloom found that the 99 deans and directors of CSWE accredited programs were cited an average of 2.9 times in 1987. In their third study of a convenience sample of four U.S. schools of social work, they found that full professors were cited more frequently in 1989, but that the rankings were mixed for associate and assistant professors. They found generally lower rates of citation on average for faculty in these four schools compared to the expert and deans samples. In their fourth study of three individual faculty, Klein and Bloom provided a more in-depth assessment of these scholars' work using statistics such as lag time that have been incorporated into the approach that is proposed below. Subsequently, Bloom and Klein (1995) studied 344 faculty from the top 13 schools identified in the Thyer and Bentley (1986) study. Overall, they found that 29.7% of these faculty had a publication listed in the Social Science Citation Index and that 76.6% of these faculty had been cited. The average rate of publication for these faculty was .56 and the average number of citations per faculty was 9.55 in 1992.

More recently, Green and Hayden (2001) examined the number of published articles and citations for the ten most productive social work faculties during the 1990-1997 period. The average faculty member in this group published 4.4 articles during the period with those articles being cited 3.27 times on average. Perhaps most revealing was that non-social work journal articles were much more frequently cited (4.22 times per non-social work vs. 1.69 times per social work article).

In summary, scholarship is a very important factor in promotion and tenure decisions. Scholars inside and outside of social work have examined ways to quantify the scholarship of individuals. This paper presents a proposal for an approach that attempts to extend the pioneering work of our colleagues. The primary goal of this paper is to stimulate discussion regarding scholarship assessment in hiring, reappointment, tenure and promotion decisions.

## *THE PROPOSED APPROACH*

How can the data available to us through the use of bibliometric techniques be used to increase the standardization of hiring, tenure and promotion decisions? Table 1 provides an example using the approach we are proposing. Most of the data for the proposed approach were obtained from the Institute for Scientific Information's Web of Science (WoS; *http://isi2.isiknowledge.com/portal.cgi/WoS*). In early 2004, the WoS provided integrated coverage of approximately 8500 leading journals from three databases (*Science Citation Expanded*, *Social Sciences Citation Index*, and *Arts & Humanities Citation Index*). These three databases can be searched separately or concurrently in the WoS. The searches below were performed using the General Search feature on all three databases concurrently, in order to capture authors' publications outside of social science venues.

The proposed approach begins with an examination of the list of articles on the candidates CV. Next one does a General Search on the WoS, covering all three databases simultaneously, using the candidate's last

TABLE 1. Demonstration of the Proposed System

| Article | n of authors | position in order of authors | MAQ | Age | N of references | Proportion of references to serials | Price Index:[1] Serials | Price Index:[1] Non-Serials | % of Synchronous self-cites[2] | Lag time (to first cite) | Persistence | Cited by self[3] | Cited by co-authors[3] | Cited by others | Total cites[3] | MAQ adjusted total cites[3] | Mean n of cites per yr. by self[3] | Mean n of cites per yr. by co-authors[3] | Mean n of cites per yr. by others | Mean n of total cites per yr.[3] | MAQ adjusted total cites per yr.[3] |
|---|---|---|---|---|---|---|---|---|---|---|---|---|---|---|---|---|---|---|---|---|---|
| Spitzer, *Holden*, Cuzzi, Rutter, Chernack & Rosenberg (2001). | 6 | 2 | .25392 | 2.5 | 52 | .48 | .44 | .15 | .15 | 1.5 | 1 | 0 | 0 | 1 | 1 | .254 | 0 | 0 | .40 | .40 | .102 |
| *Holden*, Barker, Meenaghan & Rosenberg (1999). | 4 | 1 | .53336 | 4.5 | 72 | .64 | .65 | .65 | .11 | 3.5 | 2 | 2 | 0 | 1 | 3 | 1.60 | .44 | 0 | .22 | .67 | .356 |
| *Holden*, Bearison, Rode, Rosenberg & Fishman (1999). | 5 | 1 | .516 | 4.5 | 51 | .65 | .61 | .67 | .06 | 1.5 | 3 | 2 | 0 | 5 | 7 | 3.61 | .44 | 0 | 1.11 | 1.56 | .803 |

TABLE 1 (continued)

| | n of authors | position in order of authors | MAQ | Age | N of references | Proportion of references to serials | Price Index:[1] Serials | Price Index:[1] Non-Serials | % of Synchronous self-cites[2] | Lag time (to first cite) | Persistence | Cited by self[3] | Cited by co-authors[3] | Cited by others | Total cites[3] | MAQ adjusted total cites[3] | Mean n of cites per yr. by self[3] | Mean n of cites per yr. by co-authors[3] | Mean n of cites per yr. by others | Mean n of total cites per yr.[3] | MAQ adjusted total cites per yr.[3] |
|---|---|---|---|---|---|---|---|---|---|---|---|---|---|---|---|---|---|---|---|---|---|
| Rosenberg & *Holden* (1997). | 2 | 2 | .33333 | 6.5 | 36 | .50 | .67 | .33 | .00 | 3.5 | 2 | 0 | 0 | 4 | 4 | 1.33 | 0 | 0 | .62 | .62 | .205 |
| Showers, Simon, Blumenfield & *Holden* (1995). | 4 | 4 | .06667 | 8.5 | 32 | .81 | .23 | .67 | .06 | 2.5 | 4 | 0 | 0 | 6 | 6 | .400 | 0 | 0 | .71 | .71 | .047 |
| Mailick, Holden & Walthers (1994). | 3 | 2 | .28572 | 9.5 | 27 | .67 | .22 | .44 | .00 | 2.5 | 6 | 0 | 0 | 9 | 9 | 2.57 | 0 | 0 | .95 | .95 | .271 |
| *Holden*, Rosenberg, Barker, Tuhrim & Brenner (1993). | 5 | 1 | .516 | 10.5 | 163 | .96 | .33 | .43 | .00 | 2.5 | 8 | 1 | 0 | 22 | 23 | 11.9 | .10 | 0 | 2.1 | 2.19 | 1.13 |

|  |  |  |  |  |  |  |  |  |  |  |  |  |  |  |  |  |  |  |  |  |  |
|---|---|---|---|---|---|---|---|---|---|---|---|---|---|---|---|---|---|---|---|---|---|
| Cuzzi, *Holden*, Grob & Bazer (1993). | 4 | 2 | .26668 | 10.5 | 71 | .79 | .61 | .67 | .00 | 2.5 | 2 | 1 | 0 | 3 | 4 | 1.07 | .10 | 0 | .29 | .38 | .102 |
| *Holden* (1991). | 1 | 1 | 1.0 | 12.5 | 453 | .51 | .35 | .50 | .00 | 3.5 | 10 | 9 | 0 | 38 | 47 | 47 | .72 | 0 | 3.04 | 3.76 | 3.76 |
| *Holden*, Moncher, Schinke & Barker (1990). | 4 | 1 | .53336 | 13.5 | 63 | .17 | 0 | .40 | .00 | .5 | 9 | 9 | 0 | 16 | 25 | 13.3 | .67 | 0 | 1.19 | 1.85 | .988 |
| Min. - max. | 1-6 | 1-4 | .06667-1.0 | 2.5-13.5 | 6-163 | .17-.96 | 0-.67 | .15-.67 | .00-.15 | .5-3.5 | 1-10 | 0-9 | 0 | 1-38 | 1-41 | .254-47 | 0-.72 | 0 | .22-3.04 | .38-3.76 | .047-3.76 |
| Mean | 3.8 | 1.7 | .431 | 8.3 | 55.5 | .62 | .41 | .49 | .04 | 2.4 | 4.7 | 2.4 | 0 | 10.5 | 10.7 | 8.30 | .25 | 0 | 1.06 | 1.31 | .776 |
| SD | 1.5 | .95 | .25 | 3.7 | 42.7 | .22 | .22 | .18 | .06 | .99 | 3.3 | 3.6 | 0 | 11.8 | 12.3 | 14.4 | .29 | 0 | .89 | 1.07 | 1.12 |
| Median | 4.0 | 1.5 | .425 | 9.0 | 48 | .65 | .40 | .47 | .00 | 2.5 | 3.5 | 1.0 | 0 | 5.5 | 5.5 | 2.09 | .10 | 0 | .83 | .83 | .313 |
| Total |  |  |  |  |  |  |  |  |  |  | 0 | 24 | 0 | 105 | 129 | 83.0 |  | 0 |  |  |  |

Note.

1. Price Index = the percentage of references in a paper that are not older than five years (target article publication year – referenced article publication year < 6). Price Index computed for both serials and non-serials here.

2. Synchronous self-citations as operationalized here do not include research groups listed as authors.

3. These statistics are or include types of diachronous self-citation.

4. The n for these articles does not reflect the studies used in the meta-analysis although they appear in a reference list.

5. These statistics not accurate for this author's overall work because this was a selected subset of articles.

name and first initial with a wildcard (to capture any instances when a middle initial might have been used). Then one confirms that all the articles on the CV that are in journals covered by the WoS (for that year of publication) are in fact in the databases (omissions should be reported to the WoS). Next, one records the number of authors, and the candidate's position in that array of authors.

Lindsey (1978b) proposed the *corrected quality ratio*, which combined the $n$ of publications and $n$ of citations (using a variety of adjustments). Although it has been infrequently used (e.g., Glanzel & Moed, 2002), it points to the need to understand the combination of quantity and impact of a set of articles. The *Multiple Author Qualifier* (MAQ) is our attempt to address the multiple authorship problem. Given the lack of empirical data regarding how authors in social work decide on authorship, this must be considered an initial attempt that is designed to produce discussion and refinement (this issue will be addressed in more detail in the Discussion). Beginning with the assumption that each article and each citation should only be counted once (a debatable assumption), one must next decide how each author will be credited. Table 2 details the MAQ values when using the 1/2 rule. That is, each subsequent author in the authorship list receives 1/2 of the credit of the preceding author. Other proportions are possible, yet the optimal one, if it exists, has not been determined. Using the 1/2 rule the MAQs for a four author article would be .53336, .26668, .13334 and .06667 for the first through fourth authors. These values are similar to those obtained by Wagner, Dodds and Bundy (1994) in their study of how authors value particular research tasks and determine order of authorship. While the MAQ is selectively applied in Table 2, given because of space limitations, its effect can clearly be seen. This approach may have been attempted previously although we have yet to uncover it in the literature.

Age of the article is computed by subtracting the year of publication from the current year (2003 in this case) and adding .5. The .5 was added to make the age estimate a better estimator of the age of the typical article. If an article was published in 2000 and the analysis was done in December of 2003, the age of the article might be estimated as 2003-

2000 = 3 yrs. The article could in reality be anywhere from almost four years old (1/00-12/03) to only slightly over three years old 12/00-12/03. In terms of lag time, the same applies. If an article was published in 2000 and was first cited in 2003, the lag time to citation might be estimated as 2003-2000 = 3 yrs. The time between publication and first cite could be anywhere from almost four years old (1/00-12/03) to only slightly over three years 12/00-12/03. Therefore, given that we were doing our analysis during December 2003, we added .5 years in each instance to make this a better estimator of the elapsed time.

Next the total number of references on the reference list of the article is recorded (this is provided in the WoS database). The Price Index is the proportion of references that are five years or less old (Schoepflin & Glanzel, 2001). In this approach, the Price Index for both serials and non serials is computed. The next statistic is lag time, computed as noted above. Next is persistence, which is the total number of years in which an author's work has been cited. Persistence is obviously more difficult to interpret the younger the article. The Price indices, lag times, and persistence may not be of interest to some review committees (and could be dropped from their analyses).

Aksnes (2003) states that "[a] self-citation is usually defined as a citation in which the citing and the cited paper have at least one author in common" (p. 235). He goes on to distinguish between *synchronous self-citations* (when the author cites her past work in the article that is being studied) and *diachronous self citations* (when the article that is being studied is cited by the author in one of her subsequent articles). The proposed approach focuses on citations received by target papers and therefore *diachronous self citations*–those received by the target paper from subsequent papers authored by one or more of the authors on the target paper are of most interest. Regardless, the proportion of synchronous self-citations in the target paper are also recorded (as done by Snyder & Bonzi, 1998), as they might differ from the proportion of diachronous self-citations a paper receives.

In terms of diachronous self citations–the proposed approach uses two statistics: cited by self and cited by co-authors on the original article (c.f., Fortune, 1992; Porter, 1977). Citations by others and total cites are

# BIBLIOMETRICS IN SOCIAL WORK

TABLE 2. MAQ using the rule of 1/2 (for each subsequent author) for determining portion of credit for a publication or citation.

| N of authors | Credit distribution | Formula | 1 x = |
|---|---|---|---|
| 2 | .66667 | .33333 | 2x + 1x = 1 | .33333 |
| 3 | .57144 | .28572 | .14286 | 4x + 2x + 1x = 1 | .14286 |
| 4 | .53336 | .26668 | .13334 | .06667 | 8x + 4x + 2x + 1x = 1 | .06667 |
| 5 | .516 | .258 | .129 | .0645 | .03225 | 16x + 8x + 4x + 2x + 1x = 1 | .03225 |
| 6 | .50784 | .25392 | .12696 | .06348 | .03174 | .01587 | 32x + 16x + 8x + 4x + 2x + 1x = 1 | .01587 |

Note. The credit distribution does not equal 1 due to rounding in a number of instances.

also recorded. Each of these four statistics is also adjusted for the age of the article. Cronin and Overfelt (1994) used the amount of time since first faculty appointment to adjust their raw citation counts, but noted it was a potentially flawed indicator due to the possibility of pre-appointment scholarship. The approach in the current study avoids this problem by using the age of the article to adjust the citation count for that article. This has been referred to as the citedness rate (Borgman & Furner, 2002). One issue arises from separating literal self-citation and citation by co-authors on the original paper. When a target scholar's article (article A) is cited in a subsequent article written by a group of authors that includes the target scholar and any of their co-authors on article A, this is recorded as a literal self-cite only.

Ten articles by one of the authors of this article (GH–although all of us contributed to this set of articles to some degree) are assessed in Table 1. Because this is a selection of a subset of data for demonstration purposes, two of the statistics in Table 1 are not accurate for this author (*n* of publications, *n* of publications per year studied). There were 10 articles included in the analysis or .91 articles per year for the time period studied (1990-2001). The MAQ adjusted number of articles was 4.3. All of these articles were cited and all of them were cited by individuals other then the target author (GH) or his co-authors on that article.

The typical article had four authors and this author's median position in this array was 1.5 (medians are used because of non-normal distributions). The MAQs for this set of articles ranged from .06667 to 1. This typical article was nine years old, had 48 references of which 65% were to serials. Forty percent of the references to serials and 47% of the references to non-serials were five years old or less. The proportion of synchronous self-citations ranged from .00 to .15, with a median of .00 and a mean of .04.

In terms of diachronous self citation and citation by others, the typical article was first cited two and one half years after publication and has been cited in three and one half different years after it was published. That typical article is self cited by this author one time, has not been cited by any of the co-authors on that article and is cited 5.5 times by others. Overall, this set of articles was cited 129 times (24 times by this author, 0 times by co-authors, 105 times by others). The MAQ adjusted total number of cites was 83. Three articles accounted for 74% of the citations. These three also represent three of the four oldest articles in the selected set.

Controlling for time since publication (citedness rate) it can be seen from Table 1 that the typical article is self cited by this author .1 times per year (not at all by co-authors), and is cited .83 times per year by others. The median number of MAQ adjusted total cites per year was .313.

## *PROBLEMS WITH BIBLIOMETRICS*

There are potentially problematic issues involved in the use of bibliometrics (e.g., Baker, 1990; Cnaan, Caputo & Shmuely, 1994; Garfield, 1996; 1997; Kirk, 1984; Krueger; 1993; 1999; Lindsey, 1978a; 1980; 1982; 1989; MacRoberts & MacRoberts, 1989; 1992; Narin, Olivastro & Stevens, 1994; Phelan, 1999; vonUngern-Sternberg, 2000). It is clear that citation analysis may not reflect the impact a journal article has on professionals who are reading it (but not writing and citing it).

Some of the criticisms of bibliometrics are not relevant to the approach we are proposing. For instance, this approach goes beyond the simple counting of the number of articles published and examines other aspects of the quantity and impact of a scholar's work. The approach proposed here does not restrict the set of journals studied (a critique of some studies), beyond our use of the WoS databases. Although these databases have limitations (e.g., some journals are not included and some volumes of some included journals are not included in WoS) they are the best available at this time. For individuals who publish both in and outside of social work, they allow simultaneous coverage of multiple fields.

While the *submission to publication* and *publication to first cite* time lags may have influenced some studies, any committee member with reasonable publishing experience should be aware of how these phenomena may have impacted on the candidate who is being reviewed. Long lag times (and the existence of few older publications early in one's career) do mean that the citation aspects of our approach may have more utility for later promotion decisions and the hiring of senior faculty or deans than for initial hiring or tenure decisions (c.f., Cole, 1983; cited in Garfield, 1983a).

The skewed distributions seen in many studies (e.g., many faculty rarely publish) are only a problem if those interpreting the data forget that fact. The problem with self-report data that arises in some studies is not relevant here. The self-reported data in the form of the scholar's CV is actually a benefit, because it allows the reviewers to potentially capture articles that might be missed in a WoS search due to factors such as change of institutional affiliation, change of name or initials, etc.

It also seems reasonable that citations may not be equivalent and that the types of citations vary. Some have noted that citations can occur for non-scientific reasons or they may not be positive or central to the issue being discussed. This possibility might be examined using citation context and content analyses (Garfield, 1983b) although it would probably be too resource intensive for most committees. It has also been suggested that authors may be more likely to reference work that is, for example, indexed in more commonly used databases, is more easily available to them, is written in the language they speak, or is newer, to name a few instances. In addition, authors may be referencing work that is incorrect, not referencing the best work, or not correctly referencing work. Although any or all of these possibilities may occur, we have seen no evidence that they are major problems in social work and therefore believe that they should be seen as measurement error in a non-perfect system until empirical research supports an alternative view.

Variations in citation patterns across fields, nations, time period studied or publication outlets present a potential problem for approaches such as the one proposed here. Cole (cited in Garfield, 1983a) recommends comparison of a scholar's record to "faculty members who have been promoted or granted tenure at equal caliber departments in the last several years" (p. 360). Garfield states that "[a]ll citation studies should be normalized to take into account variables such as field, or discipline, and citation practices" (1999, p. 979; c.f., Narin, Olivastro & Stevens, 1994). Yet, normalization is easier said then done (Kostoff, 2002) and given difficult problems such as this, it is clear that our approach needs substantial testing and refinement.

Another criticism is that citation analysis is narrow and shallow (e.g., Krueger, 1999). Citation analysis is a restricted view of a scholar's output (c.f., Gastel, 2001). Yet, it focuses on the output that many would argue is the most important (journal articles) and one type of impact resulting from that output. Yes, secondary analysis of any type can be trivial with no real impact on the profession. But primary analysis can be as well.

Journal coverage and technical limitations have been raised regarding the WoS. It seems logical that the level of journal coverage by the WoS will continue to increase with time, as should the capabilities of its software and interface. Similarly, alternative databases to the WoS will likely appear, allowing greater flexibility for the bibliometric researcher. Conversely, new databases will likely illuminate old problems and lead to new ones (Whitley, 2002).

Some have noted that citation analysis may be biased against high quality work that is published in very specialized journals that are read by relatively few scholars. Lindsey and Kirk (1992) found that during the 1981-89 period, although *Social Work* went to over 100,000 individuals and *Social Service Review* went out to approximately 2600, *Social Service Review* had 67% of the impact that *Social Work* had (as measured by citations in the form of impact factor scores over nine years). While this bias against work in specialized journals may exist in social work we have not found a clear demonstration of it yet.

A related concern involves these impact factor scores. A journal's impact factor is computed by "dividing the number of citations in year 3 to any items published in the journal in years 1 and 2 by the number of substantive articles published in that journal in years 1 and 2" (Saha, Saint & Christakis, 2003, p. 43). While Saha, Saint and Christakis report evidence supporting the use of impact factors as indicators of journal quality, Frank (2003) cautions us that because of inter- and intra-journal variations, citations to a scholar's articles are a better indicator of that scholar's work than the impact factor of the journals in which they are published (c.f., Furr, 1995; Garfield, 1996; 1999; Seglen, 1997; Whitehouse, 2001).

The concern that authors may be referencing themselves and thereby inflating citation rates has often been voiced. First, this critique of self-citation should not go unchallenged. We strongly agree with those who have emphasized the importance of replication in social science research (e.g., Bornstein, 1990; Neulip & Crandall, 1990; Rosenthal, 1990; Schafer, 2001). Some researchers do direct replications or replications and extensions of their prior work. In those instances it seems quite appropriate that one cite oneself in order to fully explain the research program to the reader. This should not be simply dismissed as gratuitous self-citation, but rather considered as appropriate scientific behavior. This position is indirectly supported by Klein and Bloom (1992). Second, the proposed approach distinguishes synchronous and diachronous self-citations, breaks down diachronous self citations into several categories and adjusts these statistics for the age of the article (Borgman & Furner, 2002; Cronin & Overfelt, 1994). This adds a statistic (citations by co-authors on original article) that has not, to our knowledge, been directly addressed in the literature. This dichotomization should provide review committees clarification regarding the role of self- and co-author citation. Was self-citation a major problem in this group of articles examined here? The mean proportion of synchronous self-citations in this group of articles was .04 (*Mdn = .00*). Snyder and Bonzi (1998) examined synchronous self-citations in journals in a total of six fields from the humanities, physical sciences and social sciences for the 1980-1989 period. Across all disciplines, the proportion of synchronous self-citations was .09 (.06 in economics and .07 in sociology).

Slightly under twenty percent (18.6) of the 129 citations received by the group of articles in the current study were diachronous self-citations. Aksnes (2003) studied over 45,000 science publications from Norway for the 1981-1996 period and found a diachronous self-citation rate of 21% (minimum: 17%; maximum: 31%). It appears that the rates of synchronous and diachronous self-citation observed in the articles examined here are similar to the limited normative data that is available.

Just as there are issues among authors in assigning credit for authorship (e.g., Gibelman & Gelman, 1999), researchers have discussed how multiple authorship should be handled in citation analysis. Kirk and Rosenblatt (1980) found an increase in the percentage of articles by more than one author in their study of five social work journals in the 1934-1977 period. Grinnell and Royer (1983) similarly found an increase in the 16 social work journals they examined (from initial publication through 1/1/79). Subsequently, Gelman and Gibelman (1999) found an increase in multiple authorship in four social work journals between 1973-77 and 1993-97 (c.f., Endersby, 1996; Rubin & Chang, 2003; Seaberg, 1998).

The problem created by multiple authorship in citation analysis was described over 20 years ago in social work although no consensus on the handling of the issue has been reached (e.g., Green, Hutchison & Sar, 1992; Harsanyi, 1993; Lindsey, 1978a; 1980). The following discussion assumes that a sole authored article should receive the same credit as a multiply authored article (i.e., one credit). This may not be a reasonable assumption as there is some preliminary evidence that indicates multiply authored articles are cited somewhat more frequently (e.g., Lindsey, 1978a; Oromaner, 1974).

*Normal counts (aka whole counts)*, inflate productivity estimates because multiple individuals receive full credit for a single article. *Straight counts*, which only include the article once and give all credit to the first

84    BIBLIOMETRICS IN SOCIAL WORK

author are unfair to the other authors. *Adjusted counts*, of various types have been used to award proportions of credit to coauthors (c.f., Cronin & Overfelt, 1994; Vinkler, 2000). For instance, Lindsey (1976) proposed an *adjusted total articles* measure ("summation of all of the author's articles, each divided by the number of authors," p. 802). This is the approach followed by the Council on Social Work Education in their annual report on the field and some researchers in this area (e.g., Lennon, 2002; Rothman, Kirk & Knapp, 2003). While this adjusted measure controls for the bias introduced into total number of article comparisons, it apportions credit equally to all authors of a multiply authored article. Johnson and Hull (1995) created a system which they said reflected "in part, the authors' sense of the reward system currently operative in U.S. colleges and universities" (pp. 360-1). For both journals and books/monographs, this system gave sole authors 10 points and for multiple authored articles awarded the following: first (9); second (8); third (7); fourth or more (6). While this system apportions credit relative to order of authorship, it has the same problem of over-crediting multiply authored articles (as with normal counts).

Endersby (1996) in his examination of collaborative research in the social sciences points out that whereas some fields require or tend to list authors alphabetically, the rules are clearest in psychology. While these ethical standards have been refined slightly since Endersby reviewed them, the relevant point to this discussion remains the same: "*[p]rincipal authorship and other publication credits accurately reflect the relative scientific or professional contributions of the individuals involved, regardless of their relative status*" (APA, 2002, no p., emphasis added). We believe the direction of this approach is the most appropriate. In our own experience with multiply authored articles it is clear that equivalence of contribution across authors is rarely if ever achieved.

Although resolution of the multiple authorship problem is beyond the scope of this article, we offer some alternatives to understanding this phenomenon. First, we simply recorded the number of authors on each article and the candidate's position in that array. In the summary of the articles assessed here it is easy to see that this author had from 0-5 co-authors on his articles and he typically fell between the first and second in that array. Second, we introduced the MAQ, which attempts to divide a publication or citation into proportions based on the number of authors, giving higher ranked authors a larger proportion of the credit. The single author receives one credit for each article she writes or citation she receives. The second author on a two author article receives a count of .33333 for that article, as well as a count of .3333 for each citation the article receives.

While this is a different approach from Lindsey's (e.g., 1978b; 1980) early efforts, we think it roughly echoes his and others' attempt to more equitably apportion credit for the contribution made by individuals. For instance, if normal counts of the number of publications were applied to the sample of articles examined here, a count of ten articles would have been recorded for the candidate, which overemphasizes his contribution. Using straight counts would have resulted in a total of five. Perhaps that is more reflective, but the counting of first authors only is inherently limited. Applying the MAQ to this set of articles results in a publication count value of 4.31. The MAQ does assume a single descending rate of credit (1/2) for each article, which is obviously an estimate that will not apply in each case. Yet, the MAQ maintains a value of 1 for the article (unlike normal counts); takes all authors into account (unlike straight counts), and gives greater credit to higher ranked authors (unlike the adjusted total articles approach). Obviously, computation rules other than 1/2 could be used for the MAQ (e.g., 3/4, 1/3, 1/4, etc.) and this seems to be area worth some exploration.

Some faculty reading this may be concerned that analyses such as this will lead to even more administrative intrusion upon academic freedom by facilitating increased monitoring. Our view is that the "audit culture" is already here and growing (e.g., Davenport & Cronin, 2001; Kostoff, 1996). Some faculty need to study and take control of such analyses so they are less likely to be used as weapons against faculty. Before administrators consider using bibliometrics to evaluate faculty they should remember Franck's admonition. "As a rule, however, understanding scientific facts, problems and theories is not trivial. This is why only those personally working in the respective field are competent to judge the value of a piece of scientific information" (2002, p. 6). In other words, scholars with sufficient competency to understand the applicant's content area and with sufficient competency to perform the analyses of the applicant's scholarship should have primary responsibility for hiring, retention, tenure and promotion decisions. The adoption of bibliometrics in academic employment decisions in social work merits further discussion.

## *CONCLUSION*

In summary, we began with the assertion that the assessment of scholarship is a central feature of academic life. We provided a brief background on bibliometrics, presented our proposed approach and detailed potential issues that might impact on such bibliometric analyses. The approach that was presented solves or avoids a number of the problematic issues and has the potential to add standardization to hiring, reappointment, tenure and promotion decisions. Some critics may be reading this and thinking–yes–but the problems that remain are so serious that these analyses should not be used. As Garfield (1983a; 1983b) noted years ago, and ISI still clearly states in its guidelines for citation analysis: "these methods should be used as supplement and not as replacement for careful consideration by informed peers or experts" (ISI, 2003, p. 1).

Given the importance of scholarship in the academy, it is imperative that the assessment of scholarship receives serious attention. Whether or not social work adopts part or all of the approach that has been proposed here is unimportant. What is important is that these vitally important decisions in academia become more informed, more fair.

## REFERENCES

APA (2002). Ethical principles of psychologists and code of conduct 2002. Retrieved 11/16/02 from: http://www.apa.org/ethics/code2002.html#8_12

Aksnes, D. (2003). A macro study of self-citation. *Scientometrics, 56,* 235-246.

Baker, D. R. (1990). Citation analysis: A methodological review. *Social Work Research & Abstracts, 26,* 3-10.

Baker, D. R. (1991). On-line bibliometric analysis for researchers and educators. *Journal of Social Work Education, 27,* 41-47.

Baker, D. R. (1992). A structural analysis of the social work journal network: 1985-1986. *Journal of Social Service Research, 15,* 153-168.

Baker, D. R. & Wilson, M. V. K. (1992). An evaluation of the scholarly productivity of doctoral graduates. *Journal of Social Work Education, 28,* 204-213.

Bloom, M. & Klein, W. C. (1995). Publications & citations: A study of faculty at leading schools of social work. *Journal of Social Work Education, 31,* 377-387.

Borgman, C. L. & Furner, J. (2002). Scholarly communication and bibliometrics. In B. Cronin (Ed.), *Annual Review of Information Science and Technology, 36* (pp. 3-72). Medford, NJ: Information Today.

Bornstein, R. F. (1990). Publication politics, experimenter bias and the replication process in social science research. In J. W. Neulip (Ed.) *Handbook of Replication Research in the Behavioral and Social Sciences* (pp. 71-82.). Corte Madera, CA: Select Press.

Bush, I., Epstein, I. & Sainz, A. (1997). The use of social science sources in social work practice journals: An application of citation analysis. *Social Work Research, 21, 1,* 45-56.

Cheung, K. M. (1990). Interdisciplinary relationships between social work and other disciplines: A citation study. *Social Work Research and Abstracts, 26, 3,* 23-9.

Cnaan, R. A., Caputo, R. K. & Shmuely, Y. (1994). Senior faculty perceptions of social work journals. *Journal of Social Work Education, 30,* 185-199.

Cronin, B. & Overfelt, K. (1994). Citation-based auditing of academic performance. *Journal of the American Society for Information Science, 45, 2,* 61-72.

Davenport, E. & Cronin, B. (2001). Knowledge management, performance metrics, and higher education: Does it all compute? *The New Review of Academic Librarianship, 7,* 51-65.

Endersby, J. W. (1996). Collaborative research in the social sciences: Multiple authorship and publication credit. *Social Science Quarterly, 77,* 375-392.

Euster, G. L. & Weinbach, R. W. (1983). University rewards for faculty community service. *Journal of Education for Social Work, 19,* 108-114.

Euster, G. L. & Weinbach, R. W. (1986). Deans' quality assessment of faculty publications for tenure/promotion decisions. *Journal of Social Work Education, 3,* 79-84.

Euster, G. L. & Weinbach, R. W. (1994). Faculty rewards for community service activities: An update. *Journal of Social Work Education, 30,* 317-324.

Fortune, A. E. (1992). More is not better–manuscript reviewer competence and citations: From the Past Editor-in-Chief. *Journal of Social Work Education. Research on Social Work Practice, 2*, 505-510.

Frank, M. (2003). Impact factors: Arbiter of excellence. *Journal of the American Medical Library Association, 91*, 4-6.

Franck, G. (2002). The scientific economy of attention: A novel approach to the collective rationality of science. *Scientometrics, 55, 1*, 3-26.

Furr, A. L. (1995). The relative influence of social work journals: Impact factors vs. core influence. *Journal of Social Work Education, 31*, 38-45.

Garfield, E. (1983a). How to use citation analysis for faculty evaluations, and when is it relevant? Part 1. *Current Comments, 44*, 5-13.

Garfield, E. (1983b). How to use citation analysis for faculty evaluations, and when is it relevant? Part 2. *Current Comments, 45*, 5-14.

Garfield, E. (1996). How can impact factors be improved? *BMJ, 313, 7054*, 411-413.

Garfield, E. (1997). Validation of citation analysis. *Journal of the American Society for Information Science, 48*, 962-964.

Garfield, E. (1999). Journal impact factor: A brief review. *Canadian Medical Association Journal, 161*, 979-80.

Gastel, B. (2001). Assessing the impact of investigators' work: Beyond impact factors. *Canadian Journal of Anesthesia, 48*, 941-945.

Gelman, S. R. & Gibelman, M. (1999). A quest for citations? An analysis of and commentary on the trend toward multiple authorship. *Journal of Social Work Education, 35*, 203-213.

Gibelman, M. & Gelman, S. R. (1999). Who's the author? Ethical issues in publishing. *Arete, 23, 1*, 77-88.

Gibbs, P. & Locke, B. (1989). Tenure and promotion is accredited graduate social work programs. *Journal of Social Work Education, 25*, 126-133.

Glanzel, W. & Moed, H. F. (2002). Journal impact measures in bibliometric research. *Scientometrics, 53, 2*, 171-193.

Green, R.G. (1998). Faculty rank, effort, and success: A study of publication in professional journals. *Journal of Social Work Education, 34*, 415-427.

Green, R. G., Baskind, F. R. & Conklin, B. (1995). The 1990s publication productivity of schools of social work with doctoral programs: "The times, are they a-changin?" *Journal of Social Work Education, 31*, 388-401.

Green, R. G., Baskind, F. R., Best, A. M. & Boyd, A. S. (1997). Getting beyond the productivity gap: Assessing variation in social work scholarship. *Journal of Social Work Education, 33*, 541-553.

Green, R. G., Baskind, F. R. & Bellin, M. H. (2002). Results of the doctoral faculty publication project: Journal article productivity and its correlates in the 1990s. *Journal of Social Work Education, 37*, 135-152.

Green, R. G. & Hayden, M. A. (2001). Citation of articles published by the most productive social work faculties in the 1990s. *Journal of Social Service Research, 27, 3*, 41-56.

Green, R.G., Hutchison, E. D. & Sar, B. K. (1992), Evaluating scholarly performance: The productivity of graduates of social work doctoral programs. *Social Service Review, 66*, 441-466.

Green, R. G., Kvarfordt, C. L. & Hayden, M. A. (2001). The middle years of the Decade Publication Project: 1994-97. *Journal of Social Work Education, 35*, 2, 195-202.

Grinnell, R. M. & Royer, M. L. (1983). Authors of articles in social work journals. *Journal of Social Service Research, 3/4*, 147-154.

Hargens, L. L. & Schuman, H. (1990). Citation counts and social comparisons: Scientists' use and evaluation of citation index data. *Social Science Research, 19*, 205-221.

Harrison, D. F., Sowers-Hoag, K. & Postley, B. J. (1989). Faculty hiring in social work: Dilemmas for educators of job candidates. *Journal of Social Work Education, 25*, 117-125.

Harsanyi, M. A. (1993). Multiple authors, multiple problems–bibliometrics and the study of scholarly contribution: A literature review. *Library & Information Science Research, 15*, 325-354.

Holden, G., Rosenberg, G. & Barker, K (2005a). Tracing thought through time and space: A selective review of bibliometrics in social work. *Social Work in Health Care, 41(3/4)*, 1-34.

Howard, M. O. & Howard, D. A. (1992). Citation analysis of 541 articles published in drug and alcohol journals: 1984-1988. *Journal of Studies on Alcohol, 53*, 427-434.

ISI (2003). *Interpretation.* Retrieved 1/13/04 from: http://esi-topics.com/interpreting.html

Jayaratne, S. (1979). Analysis of selected social work journals and productivity rankings among schools of social work. *Journal of Education for Social Work, 15, 3*, 72-80.

Johnson, H. W. & Hull, G. H. (1995). Publication productivity of BSW faculty. *Journal of Social Work Education, 31*, 358-368.

Jones, J. F. & Jones, L. M. (1986). Citation analysis as an approach to journal assessment in social work. *National Taiwan University Journal of Sociology, 18*, 207-219.

Kirk, S. A. (1984). Methodological issues in the comparative study of schools of social work. *Journal of Social Service Research, 7, 3*, 59-73.

Kirk, S. A. (1991). Scholarship and the professional school. *Social Work Research & Abstracts, 27*, 3-5.

Kirk, S. A. & Rosenblatt, A. (1980). Women's contributions to social work journals. *Social Work, May*, 204-209.

Kirk, S. A., Wasserstrum, K. & Miller, D. A. (1977). Publish and perish: A study of promotion and tenure in schools of social work. *Journal of Social Welfare, Winter*, 90-7.

Klein, W. C. & Bloom, M. (1992). Studies of scholarly productivity in social work using citation analysis. *Journal of Social Work Education, 28*, 291-299.

Kostoff, R. N. (1996). Performance measures for government sponsored research: Overview and background. *Scientometrics, 36*, 281-292.

Kostoff, R. N. (2002). Citation analysis of research performer quality. *Scientometrics, 53, 1*, 49-71.

Kreuger, L. W. (1993). Should there by a moratorium on articles that rank schools of social work based on faculty publications? Yes! *Journal of Social Work Education, 29*, 240-246.

Kreuger, L. W. (1999). Shallow science? *Research on Social Work Practice, 9*, 108-110.

Lennon, T. M. (2002). *Statistics on social work education in the United States: 2000.* Alexandria, VA: CSWE.

Lindsey, D. (1976). Distinction, achievement and editorial board membership. *American Psychologist, 31*, 799-804.

Lindsey, D. (1978a). *The scientific publication system in social science.* San Francisco: Jossey-Bass.

Lindsey, D. (1978b). The corrected quality ratio: A composite index of scientific contribution to knowledge. *Social Studies of Science, 8, 3*, 349-354.

Lindsey, D. (1980). Production and citation measures in the sociology of science: The problem of multiple authorship. *Social Studies of Science, 10*, 145-162.

Lindsey, D. (1982). Further evidence for adjusting for multiple authorship. *Scientometrics, 4, 5*, 389-395.

Lindsey, D. (1989). Using citation counts as a measure of quality in science: Measuring what's measurable rather than what's valid. *Scientometrics, 15*, 189-203.

Lindsey, D., & Kirk, S. A. (1992). The role of social work journals in the development of a knowledge base for the profession. *Social Service Review, 66*, 295-310.

Lindsey, D. (1999). Ensuring standards in social work research. *Research on Social Work Practice, 9*, 115-120.

MacRoberts, M. H. & MacRoberts, B. R. (1989). Problems of citation analysis: A critical review. *Journal of the American Society for Information Science, 40*, 342-349.

MacRoberts, M. H. & MacRoberts, B. R. (1992). Problems of citation analysis. *Social Work Research & Abstracts, 28*, 4.

Marsh, J. C. (1992). Should scholarly productivity be the primary criterion for tenure decisions? Yes! *Journal of Social Work Education, 28*, 132-134.

McMurty, S. L., Rose, S. J. & Cisler, R. A. (2003). Identifying and administering the most-used rapid assessment instruments. Presentation at the Seventh Annual Society for Social Work & Research Conference, Washington, DC.

Narin, F., Olivastro, D. & Stevens, K. A. (1994). Bibliometrics/theory, practice and problems. *Evaluation Review, 18, 1*, 65-76.

Neulip, J. W. & Crandall, R. (1990). Editorial bias against replication research. In J. W. Neulip (Ed.) *Handbook of Replication Research in the Behavioral and Social Sciences* (pp. 85-90). Corte Madera, CA: Select Press.

Norton, M. J. (2000). *Introductory concepts in information science.* Medford, NJ: Information Today, Inc.

Oromaner, M. (1974). Collaboration and impact: The career of multiauthored publications. *Social Science Information, 14*, 147-155.

Pardeck, J. T. (2002). Scholarly productivity of editors of social work and psychology journals. *Psychological Reports, 90*, 1051-1054.

Phelan, T. J. (1999). A compendium of issues for citation analysis. *Scientometrics, 45, 1*, 117-36.

Porter, A. L. (1977). Citation analysis: Queries and caveats. *Social Studies of Science, 7*, 257-67.

Rosenberg, G., Holden, G. & Barker, K (2005). What happens to our ideas? A bibliometric analysis of articles in *Social Work in Health Care* in the 1990s. *Social Work in Health Care, 41(3/4)*, 35-66.

Rosenthal, R. (1990). Replication in behavioral research. In J. W. Neulip (Ed.) *Handbook of Replication Research in the Behavioral and Social Sciences* (pp. 1-30). Corte Madera, CA: Select Press.

Rothman, J., Kirk, S. A. & Knapp, H. (2003). Reputation and publication productivity among social work researchers. *Social Work Research, 27*, 105-115.

Rubin, R. M. & Chang, C. F. (2003). A bibliometric analysis of health economics articles in the economics literature: 1991-2000. *Health Economics, 12*, 403-414.

Saha, S., Saint, S. & Christakis, D. A. (2003). Impact factor: A valid measure of journal quality? *Journal of the Medical Library Association, 91*, 42-46.

Sansone, F. A., Bedics, B. C. & Rappe, P. T. (2000). BSW faculty workload and scholarship expectations for tenure. *The Journal of Baccalaureate Social Work, 5, 2*, 27-46.

Schafer, W. D. (2001). Replication in field research. ERIC Digest. ERIC Identifier: ED458217. Retrieved 2/17/03 from: http://www.ericfacility.net/ericdigests/ed458217.html

Seaberg, J. R. (1998). Faculty reports of workload: Results of a national survey. *Journal of Social Work Education, 34*, 7-19.

Sellen, M. K. (1993). *Bibliometrics: An annotated bibliography, 1970-1990*. New York: G. K. Hall & Co.

Schoepflin, U. & Glanzel, W. (2001). Two decades of "Scientometrics": An interdisciplinary field represented by its leading journal. *Scientometrics, 50*, 301-312.

Seipel, M. M. (2003). Assessing publication for tenure. *Journal of Social Work Education, 39*, 79-88.

Seglen, P. O. (1997). Why the impact factor of journals should not be used for evaluating research. *BMJ, 314*. Retrieved 2/17/03 from: http://bmj.com/cgi/content/full/314/7079/497

Singer, M. [pseudonym] (2002, November 20). Collegiality and the weasel clause. *Chronicle of Higher Education*. Retrieved 11/22/02 from: http://chronicle.com/jobs/2002/11/2002112001c.htm

Snyder, H. & Bonzi, S. (1998). Patterns of self-citation across disciplines (1980-89). *Journal of Information Science, 24*, 431-435.

Thyer, B. A. & Bentley, K. (1986). Academic affiliations of social work authors: A citation analysis of six major journals. *Journal of Social Work Education, 22*, 67-73.

Twining, J. (2002). Bibliometrics: An overview. Retrieved 11/10/02 from: *http://www.du.edu/~jtwining/LIS4326/bibliometrics.htm*

Vinkler, P. (2000). Evaluation of the publication activity of research teams by means of scientometric indicators. *Current Science, 79*, 602-612.

vonUngern-Sternberg, S. (2000). Scientific communication and bibliometrics. Retrieved 11/14/02 from: *http://www.abo.fi/~sungern/comm00.htm*

Wagner, M. K., Dodds, A. & Bundy, M. B. (1994). Psychology of the scientist: Assignment of authorship credit in psychological research. *Psychological Reports, 74*, 179-187.

Whitehouse, G. H. (2001). Citation rates and impact factors: Should they matter? *The British Journal of Radiology, 74*, 1-3.

## 92 BIBLIOMETRICS IN SOCIAL WORK

Whitley, K. M. (2002). Analysis of SciFinder Scholar and Web of Science citation searches. *Journal of the American Society for Information Science and Technology, 53*, 1210-1215.

Wormell, I. (2000a). Bibliometric analysis of the welfare topic. *Scientometrics, 48*, 203-236.

Wormell, I. (2000b). Critical aspects of the Danish Welfare State–as revealed by issue tracking. *Scientometrics, 48*, 237-250.

References For Articles Used To Demonstrate Proposed Approach

Cuzzi, L. F., Holden, G. Grob, G. G. & Bazer, C. (1993). Decision making in social work: A review. *Social Work in Health Care, 18, 2*, 1-22.

Holden, G. (1991). The relationship of self-efficacy appraisals to subsequent health related outcomes: A meta-analysis. *Social Work in Health Care, 16, 1*, 53-93.

Holden, G., Barker, K., Meenaghan, T. & Rosenberg, G. (1999). Research self-efficacy: A new possibility for educational outcomes assessment. *Journal of Social Work Education, 35*, 463-76.

Holden, G., Bearison, D., Rode, D., Rosenberg, G. & Fishman, M. (1999). Evaluating the effects of a virtual environment (STARBRIGHT World) with hospitalized children. *Research on Social Work Practice, 9*, 365-82.

Holden, G., Moncher, M. S., Schinke, S. P. & Barker, K. M. (1990). Self-efficacy of children, and adolescents: A meta-analysis. *Psychological Reports, 66*, 1044-46.

Holden, G., Rosenberg, G., Barker, K., Tuhrim, S. & Brenner, B. (1993). The recruitment of research participants: A review. *Social Work in Health Care, 19*, 1-44.

Mailick, M., Holden, G. & Walthers, V. (1994). Coping with childhood asthma: Caretakers' views. *Health & Social Work, 19*, 103-11.

Rosenberg, G. & Holden, G. (1997). The role for social work in improving quality of life in the community. *Social Work in Health Care, 25*, 9-22.

Showers N., Simon, E.P., Blumenfield, S. & Holden, G. (1995). Predictors of patient and proxy satisfaction with discharge plans. *Social Work in Health Care, 22*, 19-35.

Spitzer, W., Holden, G., Cuzzi, L. C., Rutter, S., Chernack, P. & Rosenberg, G. (2001). Edith Abbott was right: Designing fieldwork experiences for contemporary health care practice. *Journal of Social Work Education, 37*, 1-12.

# Following in the Footnotes of Giants: Citation Analysis and Its Discontents

## Irwin Epstein, PhD

**SUMMARY.** Reflecting on his own personal history with bibliometrics, the author places it in the broader context of research with available information and data-mining. In so doing, he considers the utility of bibliometrics for raising new questions and its limitations for guiding decision-making. *[Article copies available for a fee from The Haworth Document Delivery Service: 1-800-HAWORTH. E-mail address: <docdelivery@haworthpress.com> Website: <http://www.HaworthPress.com> © 2005 by The Haworth Press, Inc. All rights reserved.]*

**KEYWORDS.** Available information, bibliometrics, data-mining

In three elegantly written, thoughtfully reasoned and copiously footnoted articles, Holden, Rosenberg and Barker trace the development of bibliometrics, apply it to an exploration of the relative impact of articles

---

Irwin Epstein is affiliated with the Hunter College School of Social Work, 129 East 79th Street, New York, NY 10021 (Email: iepstein@hunter.cuny.edu).

[Haworth co-indexing entry note]: "Following in the Footnotes of Giants: Citation Analysis and Its Discontents." Epstein, Irwin. Co-published simultaneously in *Social Work in Health Care* (The Haworth Social Work Practice Press, an imprint of The Haworth Press, Inc.) Vol. 41, No. 3/4, 2005, pp. 93-101; and: *Bibliometrics in Social Work* (ed: Gary Holden, Gary Rosenberg, and Kathleen Barker) The Haworth Social Work Practice Press, an imprint of The Haworth Press, Inc., 2005, pp. 93-101. Single or multiple copies of this article are available for a fee from The Haworth Document Delivery Service [1-800-HAWORTH, 9:00 a.m. - 5:00 p.m. (EST). E-mail address: docdelivery@haworthpress.com].

Available online at http://www.haworthpress.com/web/SWHC
© 2005 by The Haworth Press, Inc. All rights reserved.
doi:10.1300/J010v41n03_04

published in *Social Work in Health Care* and consider its usefulness for tenure and promotion decisions in academic settings (Holden, Rosenberg & Barker, 2005a; 2005b; Rosenberg, Holden & Barker, 2005). Although they offer multiple arguments against its applicability, their examplars imply advocacy. At a higher level of abstraction, bibliometrics may be seen as use of available information for research purposes and decision-making. At a lower level, the particular form of bibliometrics to which Holden et al. give their attention is citation analysis.

Correctly, Holden et al. trace some of the beginnings of citation analysis to a fledgling "Columbia group" of 60's doctoral students and researchers in the sociology of science who sat at the feet of a giant of modern sociology, Robert K. Merton (Cole, 2000). An encyclopedic, aloof, intimidating and, on rare occasions, intellectually playful scholar, "RKM" loved picturing himself "standing on the shoulders of giants," charting their scientific destinies. So much did he love that image, that he wrote a satirical novel under this title (Merton, 1960) in the manner of Tristam Shandy, describing a whimsical search for the origins of this oft-used metaphor.

Despite this unusual demonstration of his erudite frivolity, RKM was dead serious about the importance of understanding how social structures influence the flow of knowledge (Merton, 1957). Primarily a theoretician, rarely did he sully his hands or his scholarly explorations with quantitative data. Nonetheless, he was happy to have his young acolytes count footnotes and consider their sociological implications. Computerization was in its early stages. Citation indexes and data-bases were not available. Instead, the "group" worked with original sources, chad-vulnerable punch cards and vicious, card-devouring counter-sorters.

I know because I was a sociology doctoral student at Columbia University during this heady period. Studying under Merton and alongside the "group," I was not one of the chosen few. Nor did I choose to be. My interest in the sociology of social work was weak broth compared to the enriching potage that sociology of medicine, law and science offered. Moreover, in this crucible of structural-functional theory and analysis, the study of social problems was considered "old-school" sociology at worst and, at best, an opportunity to demonstrate the powerful and perverse "functionalist" argument that social problems persist because they contribute to societal stability.

None of this sat well with me and when I considered defecting to the University of Michigan's joint Doctoral Program in Sociology and Social Work, my advisor encouraged me to continue my studies under Richard A. Cloward, a very different sort of giant, at Columbia's School of Social Work. Formerly a student of RKM's, Cloward's groundbreaking work in delinquency theory was built on a framework supplied by Merton's *anomie* typology (Cloward & Ohlin, 1960). In turn, Merton's inspiration was the French, 19th century sociologist, Emile Durkheim (1930; 1947).

Closer to home, at the Columbia school of social work, I was told that the only way a sociologist could find employment in social work was to have a Master's degree in social work. Some things never change. Concurrently pursuing my MSW and my PhD in sociology, "RAC" became my mentor.

Stylistically and ideologically, RKM and RAC could not have been more different. Despite his humble Jewish origins, RKM (neither his real name nor initials) acted the part of the patrician scholar. The son of a Protestant minister, RAC was devoted to the role of underclass activist. Immaculately tailored and groomed, one couldn't conceive of RKM indulging in RAC's favorite lunch of Sabrett hot dogs, heavy on the mustard, onions and sauerkraut. I know because I was frequently sent out to get him his lunch. That was part of mentoring in those days and I still consider it a small price to have paid.

Wearing Fidelista fatigues and driving a Jeep long before it was hip-hop fashionable, RAC loved to rest his combat boots on seminar tables at the Carnegie Mansion, where the School of Social Work was ironically housed, and flick cigarette butts through the windows overlooking the carefully manicured garden. I shuttled between the mansion and the Columbia campus for classes. And, though RAC was my mentor, RKM left his intellectual imprint, in spite of myself.

Well before bibliometrics became bibliometrics, my interest in the sociology of social work knowledge development was conceptually shaped by RKM and ideologically informed by RAC. And while only a few subsequent papers involved counting footnotes, all were intended to raise questions about the flow of knowledge in social work and its professional/political consequences. Its first manifestation was my first published paper. Co-authored with Cloward while I was still an MSW student and reprinted several times, it is arguably my best, and without counting citations, my most influential publication. "Private Social Welfare's Disengagement From the Poor: The Case of Family Adjustment Agencies" used available agency statistics and qualitative agency interpretations of them to describe and challenge social casework's movement toward psychotherapy with middle class clients and away from provision of concrete services for the poor (Cloward & Epstein, 1965).

The explanation we offered for the movement away from the poor was the quest for professional status. Similarly, my doctoral dissertation was intended to document the negative impact of professionalization on social worker activism. Seven articles and a book later, the story is much more complex than I originally thought and fits no simple sociological paradigm (Epstein & Conrad, 1978). Two decades later, in my continuing quest to unravel its meaning, RAC and RKM still served as guides (Cheery-Reeser & Epstein, 1990, *see especially the final chapter*).

Taking my first teaching job at the University of Michigan, where behavioral alternatives to psychodynamic casework were first championed, I wrote "The Politics of Behavior Modification: the New Cool-Out Casework?" (Epstein, 1975). In that paper, I used available qualitative case examples from colleagues' published and unpublished papers, training films and classroom examples to demonstrate how behavioral techniques were used unquestioningly to promote social control of women, minorities and the poor. Seeing a training film in which a young African-American boy was taught to say "Yes Mrs. Jackson" whenever he felt angry with his teacher; hearing of a classroom example in which another faculty member proudly described his *pro bono* behavioral therapy with a depressed welfare mother by "extinguishing" her episodes of crying behavior in his office; or reading an unpublished paper by another behavior modification advocate, who trained a "promiscuous" young woman to "act like a lady, so others would treat her like a lady"; these were evidence enough for me. I suppose I was doing deconstruction before there was deconstruction. The paper was so controversial that it could only be presented at a Socialist Scholars' Conference in Wales and published in the U.K. No one in the U.S. would have it.

My fellow Michigan faculty members were not pleased. They claimed that I had used individual examples "out of context," but the real problem was too much context. They wanted "empirical evidence" that these were typical uses of the new more "scientific" alternative to psycho-dynamic casework. Rummaging in the library, I discovered a pre-coded, annotated bibliography of school-based behavior modification studies. Although not presented as a data-base, its potential for use as such was immediately apparent. It made possible a quantitative test of the social control thesis and led me to my first use of citation analysis.

Together with a student who was willing to do the footnote counting but not bring me lunch, we provided empirical evidence of the decreasing but still predominating use of "deportmental measures" (e.g., sitting still, raising one's hand before speaking, facing front, etc.) as opposed to academic performance outcomes to assess effectiveness in behavior modification studies conducted in school settings (Epstein & Hench, 1979). We even discovered that certain journals were more likely to publish aversive conditioning and control-oriented articles than others (pp. 599, 602). Not surprisingly, behavior modification journal reviewers were not pleased and roundly rejected the article. As a last resort, the paper saw the light in the *Journal of Sociology and Social Welfare*, unlikely to be read by the behavior-modification practitioners to whom it was targeted. So much for impact.

Serendipitously (a concept I learned from RKM, 1957, p. 12), in the very next issue of the same journal is published a letter to the President of Brandeis University from Norman Goroff the journal's editor protesting RAC's denial of an appointment to the Heller School "despite the unanimous recommendation of its faculty." In the letter Goroff comments that Cloward's "work on deviance has been hailed by Dr. Robert Merton as a major contribution" (Goroff, 1979, p. ii).

Frustrated in my more modest career by the perfidies of peer reviewers and the unwillingness of my Michigan colleagues to reflect on the political implications of their teachings, I took a position at Hunter College School of Social Work. Nonetheless, I kept my mid-west agency ties through work at Boysville of Michigan where along with Grasso, I promoted the development of computerized information systems for clinical and program evaluation (Grasso & Epstein, 1993). The objective was to get practitioners to use routinely available agency data in decision-making at all levels in the agency hierarchy. Together, Grasso and I convened a national conference on research utilization (Grasso & Epstein, 1992) and co-authored an article describing Boysville's practitioners' creative use of available clinical information for program and practice innovation (Epstein & Grasso, 1990). Remarkably however, this clinical information was not part of the computerized system we had spent years developing. Instead, it came from workers' case records.

In 1997, still preoccupied with the sociology of social work knowledge and practice-research utilization, I made another foray into citation analysis with two of my Hunter colleagues. This historical study of footnote sources and contents, surveyed three major social work journals from 1956 to 1992. In doing so, we discovered a significant increase in use of social science sources over time, but that this use was mediated by authors' educational credentials and organizational affiliations (Bush, Epstein & Saines, 1997). Simply stated, academically-based authors relied more heavily on social science sources. No surprise, but is it necessarily bad? Should academics be using more agency sources?

More recently, I have turned my diminishing available energies to what I call "clinical data-mining," whereby teams of agency practitioners are trained to convert their own available clinical records into quantitative or qualitative data-bases for aggregate analysis and programmatic self-reflection (Epstein & Blumenfield, 2001). I find this a remarkably effective way of engaging practitioners in learning about their own practice, in testing and refining their "practice wisdom" and in broadening their evidentiary base beyond what is conventionally thought of as "evidence-based practice." In this approach, the lessons of available research literature are integrated with those that emerge from available clinical information.

The point of this forced march through some of my own previous publications is to say that available information in general and citation analyses in particular are intriguing ways to study institutional, organizational, individual and even journal performance. Inevitably, such studies surface interesting and occasionally profound questions about practice values, norms and culture. But only if we look for them.

Unrecognized problems arise however, when studies are conducted in a political and organizational vacuum. Even worse, is when bibliometric measurements are employed narrowly and prescriptively. This is most apparent when they are used to justify invidious comparisons of one kind or another. Does this journal have more of an impact than that journal? Is one faculty member more deserving of a promotion than another? Posed in this way, the questions are utterly simplistic and their answers are subject to reification and manipulation. Consider the current effort to rank schools of social work. But that's another paper.

Returning to my Columbia school days, I'm reminded of a wonderful essay by Daniel Bell, the Marxist scholar that RKM never allowed entry into the Graduate Faculty despite his obvious brilliance, overflow lecture halls and prodigious publication record (C. Wright Mills shared a similar "outcast" status). In his article entitled "Work and Its Discontents," Bell (1960) assessed the political impact of Frederick Taylor's incredibly effective, Scientific Management approach to steel-worker productivity. Taylor honestly, if naively, thought that use of his completely empirical, a-theoretical technology would eliminate class conflict in American society. In fact, it was Taylor's fervent belief that "A fair day's work for a fair day's pay" could be arrived at through a scientific formula to which management and workers alike would naturally agree. Instead, Bell pointed out that each element in the formula could become a new and proliferating basis for union-management disagreement and negotiation (pp. 230-231).

Shifting the focal questions from the shop floor to academe, is co-authorship an indicator of collegiality or an incapacity to write solo? Is solo authorship an indicator of scholarly autonomy or the inability to work with others? Is first authorship an indicator of an exploitative exercise of authority or true intellectual leadership? Is last authorship an indicator of generous mentoring or least contribution? Formulas fail here. Probably, the answer to each begins with "it depends. . . ."

Perhaps the ultimate question is what do we mean by academic community? Indeed in lamenting the loss of "stellar" fellow faculty members to the tenure axe in favor of others, "with more production of spin than knowledge," one wonders how Holden et al. (Holden, Rosenberg & Barker, 2005a), arrived at their sense of loss? Surely not through citation analysis? And won't institutionalizing this practice produce only more "spin doctors"? It's a slippery slope from decision making "aid" to total justification.

We'll conclude our bumpy academic journey by retreating from the faculty dining room to the kitchen. As someone who delights in making use of available information, it is not surprising that I love cooking with leftovers. To do this well, one is dependent on the quality and quantity of ingredients left by others. Recipes never quite fit. Instead one is reliant on past practice, solid technique and ingenuity. Replication is rarely possible, but occasionally, just occasionally, the result is inspiring and can be shared with good friends. Even when it fails, however, it always makes for stimulating conversation. We can thank Holden, Rosenberg and Barker for doing just that.

## REFERENCES

Bell, D. (1960). Work and its discontents: The cult of efficiency in America. In *The end of ideology*, (pp. 222-262). Glencoe, IL: Free Press

Bush, I.R., Epstein, I. & Sainz, A. (1997). The use of social science sources in social work practice Journals: An application of citation analysis. *Social Work Research*, *21*(1), 45-55.

Cheery-Reeser, L. & Epstein, I. (1990). *Professionalization and activism in social work: The 60s, the 80s and the future.* New York: Columbia University Press.

Cloward, R.A. & Epstein, I. (1965). Private social welfare's disengagement from the poor: The case of family adjustment agencies. *Proceedings of the annual social work day conference.* University of Buffalo.

Cloward, R. A. & Ohlin, L.E. (1960). *Delinquency and Opportunity*. New York: Free Press.

Durkheim, E. (1947). *Division of labor in society*. Gelncoe, IL: Free Press.

Durkheim, E. (1930). *Le Suicide*. Paris: F. Alcan.

Goroff, N. (1979). Copy of a letter re Richard Cloward. *Journal of Sociology and Social Welfare, (6)5*, pp. ii.

Grasso, A.J. & Epstein, I. (Eds.) (1992). *Research utilization in the social services: Innovations for practice and administration*. Binghamton, NY: The Haworth Press, Inc.

Epstein, I. (1975). The politics of behavior therapy: The new cool-out casework? In H. Jones (Ed.), *Towards a new social work* (pp. 138-150). London: Routledge & Kegan Paul.

Epstein, I. & Blumenfield, S. (Eds.) (2001). *Clinical Data-Mining in Practice-Based Research: Social Work in Hospital Settings*. Binghamton, NY: The Haworth Press, Inc.

Epstein, I. & Conrad, K. (1978). The empirical limits of professionalization. In R. Sarri & Y. Hasenfeld (Eds.) *The management of human services*. (pp. 163-183). New York: Columbia University Press.

Epstein, I. & Grasso, A.J. (1990). Using agency-based available information to further practice innovation. In Weissman, H. (Ed.), *Serious play: Creativity and innovation in social work* (pp. 29-36). Binghamton, NY: The Haworth Press, Inc.

Epstein, I. & Hench, C. (1979). Behavior modification in the classroom: Education or social control? *Journal of Sociology & Social Welfare, 6*, 595-610.

Holden, G., Rosenberg, G. & Barker, K. (2005a). Tracing thought through time and space: A selective review of bibliometrics in social work. *Social Work in Health Care, 41* (3/4).

Holden, G., Rosenberg, G. & Barker, K. (2005b). Bibliometrics: A potential decision making aid in hiring, reappointment, tenure and promotion decisions. *Social Work in Health Care, 41*(3/4).

Merton, R.K. (1965). *On the shoulders of giants: A Shandean postscript*. New York: The Free Press.

Merton, R.K. (1957). *Social theory and social structure*. Glenoce, IL.: The Free Press. See especially Chapters 12-13 (pp. 456-508) on the sociology of knowledge.

Rosenberg, G., Holden, G. & Barker, K. (2005). What happens to our ideas? A bibliometric analysis of articles in *Social Work in Health Care* in the 1990s. *Social Work in Health Care, 41*(3/4).

# The Paradox of Faculty Publications in Professional Journals

## Robert G. Green, PhD

**SUMMARY.** The author reviews the companion papers about bibliometrics prepared for this volume and concludes that each makes a unique contribution to the growth of scholarship within the profession. However, a major practical limitation of the system advocated by the authors of these papers for faculty in schools of social work is also identified. Because only a limited number of social work faculty members produce the volume of articles required by the proposed system, the proposed system can be used currently by only a small number of schools and departments of social work. *[Article copies available for a fee from The Haworth Document Delivery Service: 1-800-HAWORTH. E-mail address: <docdelivery@haworthpress.com> Website: <http://www.HaworthPress.com> © 2005 by The Haworth Press, Inc. All rights reserved.]*

**KEYWORDS.** Bibliometrics, faculty publication, evaluating scholarship

---

Robert G. Green is Professor, School of Social Work, Virginia Commonwealth University, Richmond, VA 23284 (Email: rggreen@ucu.edu).

[Haworth co-indexing entry note]: "The Paradox of Faculty Publications in Professional Journals." Green, Robert G. Co-published simultaneously in *Social Work in Health Care* (The Haworth Social Work Practice Press, an imprint of The Haworth Press, Inc.) Vol. 41, No. 3/4, 2005, pp. 103-108; and: *Bibliometrics in Social Work* (ed: Gary Holden, Gary Rosenberg, and Kathleen Barker) The Haworth Social Work Practice Press, an imprint of The Haworth Press, Inc., 2005, pp. 103-108. Single or multiple copies of this article are available for a fee from The Haworth Document Delivery Service [1-800-HAWORTH, 9:00 a.m. - 5:00 p.m. (EST). E-mail address: docdelivery@haworthpress.com].

Available online at http://www.haworthpress.com/web/SWHC
© 2005 by The Haworth Press, Inc. All rights reserved.
doi:10.1300/J010v41n03_05

In the first of three companion articles, Holden, Rosenberg and Barker provide an excellent conceptual introduction to bibliometrics and carefully summarize the methodologies and results of previous applications of bibliometric technique and theory in the social work research literature (2005a). The authors believe that evaluations of social workers' contributions to professional journals must move beyond unsystematic and non-standardized estimates of the number of articles faculty members publish to make these evaluations fair and useful. Toward this end they suggest a set of comprehensive procedures for selecting data bases and for systematically observing the frequency with which the published articles identified are also cited in the professional literature. In so doing, the authors have crafted an approach that is unique to social workers but similar to approaches used with considerable frequency by other professions and academic disciplines.

The first paper is a prerequisite for consideration of the two subsequent papers in the series: (1) a bibliometric analysis of the 1990s articles that appeared in a designated journal (*Social Work in Health Care*) and the subsequent citations of those articles elsewhere (Rosenberg, Holden & Barker, 2005); and (2) a bibliometric decision-making aid for use by faculty committees in hiring, reappointment and promotion and tenure decisions (Holden, Rosenberg & Barker, 2005b).

The conceptual paper identifies and carefully defines the major concepts and distinctions necessary for informed discussions and analyses of contemporary social work scholarship. Holden and his colleagues organize this paper by providing distinctions between the quantity, impact and quality of scholarship, three separate but interrelated concepts that have sometimes been used interchangeably in faculty work, in faculty conversation, and in the professional literature as well. In so doing the authors reveal their extensive knowledge of bibliometrics as well as their advocacy for the use of these techniques by social work faculty and scholars. However, the paper is not merely a polemic. Unlike many discussants of bibliometrics, the authors devote a considerable amount of time and text to the disadvantages, problems and weaknesses of the method they propose. In fact, this paper may provide the single most comprehensive catalogue of the problematic nature and negative aspects of bibliometric methods in the social work literature.

In the second paper, while maintaining the same scholarly standards that characterize the first, Rosenberg, Holden and Barker (2005) evaluate, select and then apply a set of carefully reasoned bibliometric decision rules to a systematic analysis of all articles that appeared in *Social Work in Health Care* in the 1990s. Although the study provides a wealth of specific information about publication trends in this health care journal, the authors' contribution to the literature goes beyond this descriptive function. Indeed, in tandem with the former paper this article provides a template for continuing knowledge development about social work scholarship through the use of existing data bases. To develop a more informed, broader look at the profession's scholarship, subsequent bibliometric analyses will benefit from replicating this study using social work journals, designated subsets of social work journals, and specific non-social work journals in which social workers publish.

The third paper in this series also encourages and facilitates the continuing application of bibliometric methods in social work, in this instance by focusing specifically on the publications and citations of those faculty members who have developed a record of publication and whose articles have been cited by others (Holden, Rosenberg & Barker, 2005b). To provide a basis for peer evaluation of the publications and article citations of these successful social work scholars, the authors propose the use of the Web of Science, clearly the most comprehensive and systematically updated data base available. They also provide a list of 21 different variables pertinent to the description and subsequent citation of each article published by the faculty member being evaluated. In addition, to test and facilitate use of the proposed system as a whole, the authors also provide the actual data that resulted from the evaluation of 10 articles published by the senior author.

Variable choices and specific bibliometric decision rules for data collection are incorporated into the authors proposed system *only* after a full review and consideration of measurement options previously advocated or used in earlier studies, and *only* after providing a clear rationale for their choice. These decision rules include methods for determining publication dates and the elapsed time since those publication dates, methods for proportionately attributing authorship and subsequent citations of multiple authored articles, and a procedure for identifying, controlling and accounting for different types of self citation.

A major limitation of the proposed system, however, is that it is applicable only to the evaluation of a limited number of social work faculty members–those who are successful scholars–and can therefore be used by committees in only a small number of schools and departments. As the authors indicate, their system pertains only to "individuals who have amassed a body of scholarship that can be assessed" and that the system "will likely not be relevant for hiring at the assistant professor level" (Holden, Rosenberg & Barker, 2005b). And, as their review of the literature demonstrates, the publication in professional journals is not a frequent and re-occurring event for faculty at most schools of social work. Unfortunately, this is even true for a substantial number of faculty members at colleges and universities where scholarship is a *major* expectation.

In spite of the relatively robust rates of publication in the 1990s by faculty members of a few research intensive schools of social work, data collected for the Decade Publication Project suggests that the typical faculty member of these 61 doctoral degree granting graduate programs published (in professional journals) infrequently over the course of the decade. The mean number of articles published each year for all 61 faculties was only 0.28, just a little more than one article every 4 years (Green, Baskind & Bellin, 2002). Surprisingly, substantial numbers of faculty members *did not publish a single article* in a professional journal during the 1990s. It is reasonable to assume, therefore, that the publication paucity which characterizes the schools with doctoral programs is even more evident and prevalent among the non-doctoral degree granting schools and departments as well.

Consequently, the majority of social work evaluation committees might find *partial application* of the system presented by Holden, Rosenberg and Barker–merely counting a faculty member's publications in selected refereed journals–a considerably more parsimonious, less labor intensive and more useful way of evaluating the majority of social work faculty members' scholarship in professional journals. However, applying the methods suggested by Holden and his colleagues for standardizing data bases and for identifying and attributing authorship in the case of multi-authored articles should be of considerable use to these schools and to the profession. The use of this more limited aspect of the system will increase the reliability and fairness of evaluations within schools as well as provide for more precise comparisons across faculty units.

The lack of robustness in the publication rates of social work faculty members should not be taken as an indicator of the importance of publication among social work faculty. Indeed, as Holden and his colleagues point out, recent survey data suggests that full-time social work faculty continue to consider publication of articles as *the most important* of all indicators of scholarship (Seipel, 2003). And, the total number of journal articles published by each of the 61 doctoral faculties during the 1990s was strongly correlated ($r = .78$) with the academic quality ratings of MSW programs completed at the end of the decade (1999) for the *US NEWS* rankings by social work deans, directors and senior faculty. Further analysis of these data (multiple regression) revealed that this raw publication count was the *only* correlate of perceived academic quality for these schools when the influences of the age or longevity of the university, the school and the doctoral program as well as the size of the faculty, the university and the student body of each school were evaluated simultaneously (Green, Baskind & Bellin, 2002).

Because the first wave of data collection for the second decade (2000-2009) of the Decade Publication Project and the 2004 *US News* academic quality ratings of the graduate schools of social work are now available, we also correlated the total number of publications for faculties of each of these same schools between January 2000 and September 2003 with the academic quality ratings that social work deans, program directors and senior faculty members completed for *US News* in the fall of 2003. The results for this additional more current analysis so far in the 2000s were similar to those obtained for the 1990s. The zero order correlation between academic quality ratings and the number of publications was .85.

*108*        *BIBLIOMETRICS IN SOCIAL WORK*

Although social work faculty members publish infrequently, they continue to view faculty publication as the strongest available indicator of the academic quality of graduate programs. The former may be bad news for the profession and social work education in the 2000s, but the latter is certainly good news.

## REFERENCES

Green, R. G., Baskind, F. R. & Bellin, M.H. (2002). Results of the doctoral faculty publication project: Journal article productivity and its correlates in the 1990s. *Journal of Social Work Education, 37,* 135-152.

Holden, G., Rosenberg, G. & Barker, K. (2005a). Tracing thought through time and space: A selective review of bibliometrics in social work. *Social Work in Health Care, 41* (3/4), 1-35.

Holden, G., Rosenberg, G. & Barker, K. (2005b). Bibliometrics: A potential decision making aid in hiring, reappointment, tenure and promotion decisions. *Social Work in Health Care, 41* (3/4), 67-92.

Rosenberg, G., Holden, G., & Barker, K. (2005). What happens to our ideas? A bibliometric analysis of articles in *Social Work in Health Care* in the 1990s. *Social Work in Health Care, 41* (3/4), 35-66.

Seipel, M.O. (2003). Assessing publication for tenure. *Journal of Social Work Education, 39,* 79-90.

# Politics of Personnel
# and Landscapes of Knowledge

## Stuart A. Kirk, PhD

**SUMMARY.** This is a commentary on three articles on bibliometrics in social work that appear in this volume. I argue that bibliometrics can make many contributions to the study of the structure and evolution of social work's knowledge base, but it cannot completely remove subjectivity in the evaluation of the scholarship of individual faculty, where legitimate differences of professional opinion will remain. *[Article copies available for a fee from The Haworth Document Delivery Service: 1-800-HAWORTH. E-mail address: <docdelivery@haworthpress.com> Website: <http:// www.HaworthPress. com> © 2005 by The Haworth Press, Inc. All rights reserved.]*

**KEYWORDS.** Bibliometrics, citaton analysis, faculty evaluation

---

Stuart A. Kirk is Professor, Department of Social Welfare, School of Public Affairs, 3250 Public Policy Building, UCLA, Los Angeles, CA 90095-1656 (E-mail: kirk@ucla.edu).

[Haworth co-indexing entry note]: "Politics of Personnel and Landscapes of Knowledge." Kirk, Stuart A. Co-published simultaneously in *Social Work in Health Care* (The Haworth Social Work Practice Press, an imprint of The Haworth Press, Inc.) Vol. 41, No. 3/4, 2005, pp. 109-116; and: *Bibliometrics in Social Work* (ed: Gary Holden, Gary Rosenberg, and Kathleen Barker) The Haworth Social Work Practice Press, an imprint of The Haworth Press, Inc., 2005, pp. 109-116. Single or multiple copies of this article are available for a fee from The Haworth Document Delivery Service [1-800-HAWORTH, 9:00 a.m. - 5:00 p.m. (EST). E-mail address: docdelivery@haworthpress.com].

Available online at http://www.haworthpress.com/web/SWHC
© 2005 by The Haworth Press, Inc. All rights reserved.
doi:10.1300/J010v41n03_06

Professor Smith: "The candidate should be granted tenure; she has published 12 articles."

Professor Jones: "We should expect more."

Professor Smith: "But quantity alone isn't that important. Her articles are quite good."

Professor Jones: "Not good enough."

## INTRODUCTION

I don't recall what motivated me decades ago to go to the university library's reference room and use the Social Science Citation Index for the first time. None of my social work colleagues, as far I as I knew, had ever heard of it. I remember pouring over the large annual tomes containing lists of references contained in published articles and lists of citations made to published articles. Perusing these arcane reference books was peering at the inchoate raw underbelly of academic scholarship, but I didn't perceive this mountain of information as "data," because of the amount of labor involved in using the volumes. Computerized databases have changed all that. Libraries now provide direct access to the databases of the Institute for Scientific Information, which gathers, organizes and makes available the citation indexes. New topics and entire fields of inquiry have resulted from these electronic capacities, as was noted in a recent colloquium of the National Academy of Sciences (Shiffrin & Borner, 2004).

## BIBLIOMETRICS

Bibliometrics is one strand of this information retrieval explosion, and Holden, Rosenberg and Barker (Holden, Rosenberg & Barker, 2005a; 2005b; Rosenberg, Holden & Barker, 2005) in their three informative and well-argued articles are introducing and providing illustrations of some of the potential uses of these new capacities for gauging social work articles. The objectives of each of their articles are specific and different. In one, "Tracing thought through time and space," they summarize the uses, methodological problems, and findings from bibliometrics studies that have appeared in social work since the 1970s. They note that past studies have found that few social workers publish, editorial boards are relatively weak, and, in general the scholarly infrastructure of social work is not as robust as in academic disciplines. In the second, "What happens to our ideas?" they report findings from their exploratory study of the characteristics of the most heavily cited articles from one specialty journal. In the third, they propose a method of evaluating the scholarship of individual faculty. They illustrate this method with data gathered about their own articles and describe how bibliometric methods should be used to assess the quantity and impact of a person's publications in personnel decisions.

By producing this set of papers, they have done a service to social work. They succinctly summarize a scattered literature; they provide a user-friendly introduction to the methods, struggles and past controversies involving bibliometrics in social work; and they have given us three new citations where we can now send students or faculty who want to get up-to-speed on this topic. In addition, as a bonus, the papers are written in an accessible style and address most of the concerns that might be raised about the limits of their work.

But–there is always a but–when new researchers turn to these papers for an orientation to the topic, there are other considerations that they need to recognize. Space permits me to mention just two. One has to do with the evaluation of faculty. The second with tracing ideas.


## EVALUATION OF FACULTY

Holden, Rosenberg and Barker (2005b) knew there would be sparks about their faculty evaluation proposal and they effectively doused most of them. Their goal is unassailable. They want faculty hiring and promotion decisions to be "fair and equitable"(abstract), to be "more informed, more fair," to be "free from bias." They claim, without providing evidence, that fairness ". . . is not what happens in untold instances" and that with personnel evaluations the "level of subjectivity . . . can be distressing." Actually evidence is probably not needed to persuade colleagues of the veracity of these conclusions because it confirms many professors' own perceptions. In fact, as I was beginning to work on this commentary, a recent doctoral graduate now on the faculty at a major research university told me, without my solicitation, that she was surprised by how murky, unpredictable and vaguely "political" personnel decision-making seemed to be.

Research universities spend an embarrassingly wasteful amount of time and resources in peer review processes, in which there are elaborate layers of review at the department, school and university level. How is it that this process can be so often perceived as "subjective" when multiple sources of evidence are acquired, where the opinions of both insiders and outsiders are consulted, and in which everyone is on heightened alert to avoid even the taint of race, gender, sexual orientation or age bias? And, more to the point, would the Holden et al. (2005b) carefully calibrated indices remedy this?

If the evaluations of faculty were straightforward and could be handled by objective indicators, universities long ago would have adopted them and eliminated the expensive review procedures. Faculty often agree in the abstract on some general principles about what constitutes good scholarship, good teaching or good service. Their consensus, however, frequently vanishes when it comes to applying these principles to a specific individual at a particular point in time, unless the candidate is an outlier with a sterling or abysmal record. In addition, over and above the actual performance of the candidate, the faculty legitimately consider the school's long-term curriculum needs, the need for faculty diversity, and a host of other relevant local considerations that may have little to do with the quality of the scholarship. University review procedures are complicated and multi-layered *precisely because there often is disagreement* about the application of these general principles to the evaluation of a specific individual. This problem is one of the motivations behind Holden et al.'s proposal.

As personnel decisions wind their way through these murky processes, there are frequently differences of opinion about the candidate's performance, the relevant contextual considerations and other matters. When these differences in peer review are expressed in faculty votes, the result is "political" by definition. Voting is one of the processes we have chosen to manage differences of opinion in university faculty evaluation and elsewhere. There are other methods of making decisions, but they generally aren't as appealing.

In one of the true instances of faculty egalitarianism, every faculty member sooner or later gets to experience being in the minority, that is, of voting in the minority either for a candidate who fails to succeed or against a candidate who gains the promotion anyway. At these moments, when one's own precious wisdom about the merits of a candidate is rejected, it is very tempting to conclude that the decision was based on others' subjectivity, unfairness or bias. Of course, when on the winning side, one concludes that fairness won out. This, I think, explains why so many share this vague sense that personnel decisions are sometimes unfair. Holden et al. clearly want to promote more fairness and reduce bias, but they need to be careful not to confuse legitimate differences of professional opinion with bias or irrelevant subjectivity.

Should we strive for more objectivity and fairness? Absolutely. Are there really instances in which faculty and the quality of their scholarship have been unfairly judged, where bias and invidious subjectivity have really intruded? Certainly. Will the Holden et al. methods help? Here, I'm less certain, because their various objective indicators, such as the "MAQ adjusted total cites," thoughtfully developed as they are, do not speak for themselves. The meaning, interpretation, relevance and application of these indices in any given instance still must come from the professional judgment of colleagues. For example, what is a personnel committee to make of the fact that a candidate's MAQ adjusted total cites per year is .77, or 1.77 or 2.77? Their usefulness is only in relation to some standard that may provide some meaning. We don't yet have such standards and so we are left with ambiguities, much as we are when we try to "objectively" assess student evaluations of teaching or service to the university. In addition, any one piece of information, whether about teaching or scholarship, is often overwhelmed by the complexities of the candidate's full record and the need to consider contextual factors, such as the current needs of the school, unique aspects of the person's work and role in the program, the scholarship's contribution in the subfield, the evolutionary stage of the subfield, and the likely trajectory of that person's research.

There are several circumstances, however, where the careful counting proposed by Holden et al. may be very useful in improving personnel outcomes. These are instances where there is, in fact, blatant bias on the part of some of the candidate's colleagues who may be claiming incorrectly either that the candidate's truly mediocre work is outstanding or that a candidate's truly outstanding work is at best mediocre. In these instances of sharp disagreements among colleagues about the merits of the scholarship, university review committees and administrators often have difficulty deciphering the validity of contradictory claims. Under these circumstances, objective, independent indicators of the sort that Holden et al. propose could serve as very useful gauges of the quantity and quality of the work and a guard against gross unfairness and subjectivity.

Certainly, the more information that is available, the better for everyone. The more objective and independent that information, as Holden et al. suggest, the better. But in the gurgling caldron of faculty evaluation, I am less persuaded that citation rate scores are likely to eliminate much subjectivity. I can too easily imagine that the same citation score that will be used by the candidate's supporters as evidence that the work is cited, will be used by the detractors as evidence that the work is not cited enough. We currently see similar differences of opinion when faculty discuss the worth of an article or the quality of the journal it appears in. So, we may be left in the end confronted with differences of professional opinion about the extent to which bibliometric indices provide an adequate measure of the candidate's scholarship. Because of this, there may be accusations of illegitimate subjectivity no matter what the outcome turns out to be. Nevertheless, any attempt to introduce more objectivity should be welcomed.

In my opinion, the kind of bibliometrics discussed by Holden et al. are potentially most useful, not in the assessment of the value of any one scholar's work, but in comparative studies of institutions, groups of faculty, journals and studies of historical trends. But even with aggregate comparative studies, a caution is needed.

## TRACING IDEAS

The caution is not to conflate articles with ideas. The paper, "What happens to our ideas?" (Rosenberg et al., 2005), is a catchy title, but not at all about tracing ideas; it is about citation patterns to specific articles. Citation patterns describe one type of web of connections in a body of literature, but they don't describe its intellectual content. Article citation, at best a proxy for the recent usefulness of an article, is not about ideas themselves. The distinction is substantively important. One could conduct an elaborate study of citation patterns without even describing the nature of any central idea or contribution.

Bibliometric methods in social work are still scratching the surface of the field's knowledge base. Can we use these evolving bibliometric methods to identify the core or influential ideas in social work and trace their evolution? For example, can we use bibliometrics to learn more about the evolution of ideas such as person-in-environment, harm reduction, child abuse, social justice, diversity, welfare-to-work, post traumatic stress disorder, evidence-based practice, or empowerment? Although studies of the history of ideas have and can be conducted without bibliometric methods, can computerized databases of the periodical literature deepen our understanding of the history, nature and direction of our professional knowledge base?

The use of bibliometrics to focus on any one individual's work or any single article is to focus on the insignificant (unless of course the person is the likes of Freud or Einstein). Every article is a small seed dropped on an unforgiving terrain. The majority never germinates; a few survive for a season or two. Only a rare seed, blessed by its natural hardiness and favored by unique historical circumstances, flourishes and eventually stimulates the growth of a lush landscape that is enjoyed for a generation. We need more studies of these intellectual landscapes in social work. Perhaps bibliometrics and Holden et al.'s papers can help move us in that direction. If so, it will produce a windfall of citations to their work.

## REFERENCES

Holden, G., Rosenberg, G. & Barker, K (2005a). Tracing thought through time and space: A selective review of bibliometrics in social work. *Social Work in Health Care, 41*(3/4), 1-34.

Holden, G., Rosenberg, G. & Barker, K (2005b). Bibliometrics: A potential decision making aid in hiring, reappointment, tenure and promotion decisions. *Social Work in Health Care, 41*(3/4), 67-92.

Rosenberg, G., Holden, G. & Barker, K (2005). What happens to our ideas? A bibliometric analysis of articles in *Social Work in Health Care* in the 1990s. *Social Work in Health Care,* 41(3/4).

Shiffrin, R. M., & Borner, K. (2004). Mapping knowledge domains. *Proceedings of the National Academy of Sciences, 101* (supplement 1), 5183-5185.

# Bibliometrics:
# The Best Available Information?

### Waldo C. Klein, PhD, MSW
### Martin Bloom, PhD

**SUMMARY.** This commentary raises significant cautions related to inherent shortcomings in the use of bibliographic analytic technology, and in particular its use in substantive decision making around promotion and tenure. Questions are raised concerning the continued use of scholarly energy for bibliometric analysis of subtly different settings. The recommendation is offered that future efforts in bibliometrics must target methods to reduce methodological shortcomings. These include clarifying the metric used to "count" sole/multiple authorship, and to evaluate the "merit" of manuscripts as well as journals in which they appear. Finally, the fundamental meaning of the information produced in these analyses (i.e., the

---

Waldo C. Klein (E-mail: Waldo.Klein@uconn.edu) and Martin Bloom (E-mail: Martin.Bloom@uconn.edu) are affiliated with the School of Social Work, University of Connecticut, 1798 Asylum Avenue, West Hartford, CT 06117.

[Haworth co-indexing entry note]: "Bibliometrics: The Best Available Information?." Klein, Waldo C., and Martin Bloom. Co-published simultaneously in *Social Work in Health Care* (The Haworth Social Work Practice Press, an imprint of The Haworth Press, Inc.) Vol. 41, No. 3/4, 2005, pp. 117-121; and: *Bibliometrics in Social Work* (ed: Gary Holden, Gary Rosenberg, and Kathleen Barker) The Haworth Social Work Practice Press, an imprint of The Haworth Press, Inc., 2005, pp. 117-121. Single or multiple copies of this article are available for a fee from The Haworth Document Delivery Service [1-800-HAWORTH, 9:00 a.m. - 5:00 p.m. (EST). E-mail address: docdelivery@haworthpress.com].

Available online at http://www.haworthpress.com/web/SWHC
© 2005 by The Haworth Press, Inc. All rights reserved.
doi:10.1300/J010v41n03_07

*validity of the measure) must be clearly presented in order for it to be credibly used. [Article copies available for a fee from The Haworth Document Delivery Service: 1-800-HAWORTH. E-mail address: <docdelivery@haworth press.com> Website: <http://www.HaworthPress.com> © 2005 by The Haworth Press, Inc. All rights reserved.]*

**KEYWORDS.** Bibliometrics, citation analysis, promotion and tenure

These three papers provide the reader with a reasonable snapshot of bibliometric methods in social work scholarship; with the strengths, as well as the warts and blemishes in fairly plain view. One paper reviews the literature of these methods and in doing so identifies major issues–positive and negative–in their past use. A second applies biblio- metric methods to review a decade's worth of publications in one selected journal. The third proposes the application of bibliometrics as a tool in making tenure and promotion decisions. The authors of these papers clearly encourage the use of these methods, even as they are aware of significant limitations.

We, too, see the possible value in these methods. We believe that decision making in areas such as social work scholarship for school ranking and promotion and tenure should be guided by the *"best available information."* To that end, bibliometrics *may* offer a component of decision-making information. However, we believe that significant cautions are in order for at least two fundamental reasons.

First, as Holden, Rosenberg and Barker point out in these papers, there are many shortcomings inherent in this emerging technology (Holden, Rosenberg & Barker, 2005a; 2005b; Rosenberg, Holden & Barker, 2005). At what point do their identified shortcomings become too serious or too numerous to offset the presumed value imparted by bibliometric techniques? A hallmark of the *best available information principle* is that it involves a precise understanding of what is being measured. For example, these authors claim to assess "impact." And yet, even as they share that bibliometrics offers but one indicator, they are prompt in operationalizing this construct in terms of citations to a given work. The results of this operationalization may be an instance of what Donald Campbell has termed the "unmitigated disaster [of] the advice to employ designated operational definitions for theoretical terms"

(Campbell & Russo, 1999, p. 167). This process results in the richness of the term "impact" being reduced to an enumeration of citations, and citations themselves reflect unclear and even dubious meaning. We fear that we may be coming to know more and more about less and less! With regard to the making of promotion and tenure decisions generally, Kirk, Wasserstrum and Miller (as cited in Holden, Rosenberg & Barker, 2005a) suggest that we "have developed refined methods of applying vague generalities." Bibliometrics may simply be extending our refinement of vague generalities to new heights.

Second, in light of the acknowledged shortcomings, is it appropriate for the profession to spend limited scholarly energy and resources on continued application of the methods to subtly different study settings–academic units, journals, individual scholars? When bibliometric methods are used to precisely rank schools, individuals, journals or anything else, we need to more fully address the underlying question: What specifically are we trying to evaluate? Given the conceptual confusion that is apparent in the meaning of these counts, we really must ask the essential question– "What does it mean?" Does the metric really matter? Duncan Lindsey (as cited in Holden, Rosenberg & Barker, 2005b) recognized a decade and a half ago that while citation counts in the extremes (no citations and those in the very highest ranges) are probably indicative of *something*, those in the middle–and we would expect that this captures the great majority of individuals–probably do not distinguish anything among scholars. As others (cited in these papers) have suggested, perhaps a moratorium on papers such as these is in order.

But yet, if we are in search of the *best available information*, further development of these methods may be useful. Perhaps a balance can be struck by focusing all bibliometric scholarly activity on the development of the method itself, rather than on the application of the method. But the value served should be on the enhancement of a promising technology. Having recognized many of the limitations that have been present in past bibliometric efforts, the goal should be on eliminating these methodological and philosophical stumbling blocks. This is perhaps the intent of Holden, Rosenberg and Barker when they note that "bibliometrics is in a

## 120            *BIBLIOMETRICS IN SOCIAL WORK*

process of evolution" (Holden, Rosenberg & Barker, 2005b). If so, this goal needs to be made much more clearly.

In the meantime, application of bibliometric methods to questions of substance creates troubling issues. Nowhere is this more clearly illustrated than in the process of tenure and promotion review. First, because of the time lags in publication and citation, these methods may not be at all applicable for most junior faculty seeking their first tenure appointment. In any case, while a strong bibliometric record may be solid evidence in support of one's tenure decision, the lack of same may not be indicative of a scholarly void. One's scholarly record may take different forms, and the appreciation and analysis of these multiple forms is not easily reduced to a formulaic assessment. Likewise, in hiring decisions, current bibliometric procedures may offer the basis for identifying one kind of strength among candidates, but search committees are generally interested in reaching a decision that maximizes a number of competing characteristics and as with tenure consideration, the lack of a strong bibliometric record cannot be taken of evidence of a scholarly void.

## *CONCLUSION*

Bibliometric analysis of schools or scholars may indeed offer one opportunity to seek the *best available information* for application in a variety of settings. However, in order for us to ensure that this is the case, future attention must be targeted on methods to reduce the recognized shortcomings involved in the methods. While some of these relate to technical aspects of bibliometrics (i.e., the use of specific data bases, comparisons across time or discipline, the correlation between citations and the circulation of the publishing journal, etc.), others are more philosophical–and we believe fundamental. These include issues such as the metric to be applied to sole/multiple authorship, the relative merit (influence? impact?) of the article itself in whatever in whatever journal in which citations appear, the legitimacy of self-citation, and ultimately, determination and agreement on exactly what is intended by the enumerations involved in bibliometrics–the validity question. If these issues can be successfully resolved, bibliographic methods have the potential of heightening one component of the *best available information principle* with respect to scholarly activity. If they cannot, bibliographic methods will become increasingly recognized as an "answer"– in search of a question.

## REFERENCES

Campbell, D. & Russo, M. J. (1999). *Social experimentation*. Thousand Oaks, CA: Sage.

Holden, G., Rosenberg, G. & Barker, K (2005a). Tracing thought through time and space: A selective review of bibliometrics in social work. *Social Work in Health Care*, *41*(3/4), 1-34.

Holden, G., Rosenberg, G. & Barker, K (2005b). Bibliometrics: A potential decision making aid in hiring, reappointment, tenure and promotion decisions. *Social Work in Health Care*, *41*(3/4), 67-92.

Rosenberg, G., Holden, G. & Barker, K (2005). What happens to our ideas? A bibliometric analysis of articles in *Social Work in Health Care* in the 1990s. *Social Work in Health Care*, *41*(3/4), 35-66.

# Bibliometrics and Social Work:
# A Two-Edged Sword
# Can Still Be a Blunt Instrument

Jan Ligon, PhD
Bruce A. Thyer, PhD

**SUMMARY.** In order to improve the productivity and impact of social work scholarship, the profession must look beyond bibliometrics to other issues that must be considered. These include the lag time between acceptance and publication of articles, the quality of peer review experienced by social work authors, and the overabundance of journals being published in social work. *[Article copies available for a fee from The Haworth Document Delivery Service: 1-800-HAWORTH. E-mail address: <docdelivery@haworthpress.com> Website: <http://www.HaworthPress.com> © 2005 by The Haworth Press, Inc. All rights reserved.]*

---

Jan Ligon is affiliated with the School of Social Work, Georgia State University. Bruce A. Thyer is affiliated with the School of Social Work, Florida State University.

Address correspondence to: Jan Ligon, PhD, School of Social Work, College of Health and Human Services, University Plaza, Georgia State University, Atlanta, GA 30303-3083 (E-mail: ligon@gsu.edu).

[Haworth co-indexing entry note]: "Bibliometrics and Social Work: A Two-Edged Sword Can Still Be a Blunt Instrument." Ligon, Jan, and Bruce A. Thyer. Co-published simultaneously in *Social Work in Health Care* (The Haworth Social Work Practice Press, an imprint of The Haworth Press, Inc.) Vol. 41, No. 3/4, 2005, pp. 123-128; and: *Bibliometrics in Social Work* (ed: Gary Holden, Gary Rosenberg, and Kathleen Barker) The Haworth Social Work Practice Press, an imprint of The Haworth Press, Inc., 2005, pp. 123-128. Single or multiple copies of this article are available for a fee from The Haworth Document Delivery Service [1-800-HAWORTH, 9:00 a.m. - 5:00 p.m. (EST). E-mail address: docdelivery@haworthpress.com].

Available online at http://www.haworthpress.com/web/SWHC
© 2005 by The Haworth Press, Inc. All rights reserved.
doi:10.1300/J010v41n03_08

KEYWORDS. Social work scholarship, social work authors, peer reviewed journals, bibliometrics

Holden, Rosenberg, and Barker provide social workers with a comprehensive review and analysis of bibliometrics in its various forms and offer some interesting, if not disappointing, observations about social work and scholarship (Holden, Rosenberg & Barker, 2005a; 2005b; Rosenberg, Holden & Barker, 2005). Indeed this approach to assessing scholarship can apparently be traced to a 1927 analysis of a chemistry journal (Garfield, 1972). As Holden, Rosenberg and Barker (2005a) so aptly note, a plethora of articles using bibliometrics have been published over the years in the social work literature, presumably to shed new light on the profession's scholarship.

As noted by Holden, Rosenberg and Barker (2005b), systematic analysis of the work of academics is on the increase and social work joins many other disciplines in undertaking such investigations. For example, The American Society of Pediatric Neurosurgeons reviewed over 1,800 citations in their field's professional journals and found that 75% of their members published less than half of their work in their discipline-specific journals (Dias, 1998), paralleling a similar pattern of publishing in non-disciplinary journal outlets among social work academics (Green, Bellin & Baskin, 2002). The field of criminal justice has published numerous articles that examine the institutional productivity of authors (Sorensen, 1994; Taggart & Holmes, 1991), the effect of gender on productivity (Stack, 2002), and the historical contributions of African American scholars in early criminology texts (Gabbidon & Greene, 2001). Another study found that those who are most cited in criminology journals are not the same as those most cited in criminology textbooks (Wright, 2002). In psychology, a study of the most cited authors in introductory psychology texts found Sigmund Freud to be the most cited, with an average of 28 pages per text, and more than double that devoted to Jean Piaget, the next most cited author (Griggs & Proctor, 2002). For decades, the works of B. F. Skinner have been cited hundreds of times annually, with no diminuation evident over time (Thyer,

1991). Thus within criminology and psychology, as in many other fields, scholarship involving bibliometric analysis is a thriving industry, and can be seen as an valid component of the sociology of one's disciplinary science.

But is all this effort really useful? A Web of Science search (*http:// isi4.isiknowledge.com/portal.cgi*) finds that Ligon, Thyer, and Dixon (1995) has been cited twelve times, being cited every year except 2000 from 1998-2003, and has been self-cited twice. Is this then a "quality" article and has it had an "impact?" (Most published articles are never cited at all, ever!) While Holden, Rosenberg and Barker (2005b) make a case that there are ways to answer these questions, others have noted "the inherent difficulties in trying to quantify an essentially intangible concept–the relative quality and importance of research" (Sims & McGhee, 2003, p. 22). Yet the fact that Thyer et al. (1985) has been cited 124 times over its lifetime is a compelling argument that this is a more meaningful contribution to scientific discourse than, say, Keopke and Thyer (1985), which has been cited only 3 times. Complicating such a judgement is the possibility that, perhaps, Thyer et al. (1985) made particularly outrageous or unjustifiable claims (we do not believe this to be the case, but are making a purely hypothetical argument) which more competent scholars have been busy commenting on and re-futing ever since. Does such a flurry of activity engendered by a notori-ous article constitute a constructive contribution to science? We also note with wry humor that the social work programs rated most highly in publication productivity studies such Ligon, Thyer and Dixon (1995) often cite this fact in their recruitment and publication relations media! Is this a constructive outcome of an article?

More attention should be paid to improving the relatively low level of publication rates characteristic of many social work faculty, relative to scholars in other disciplines (Thyer & Polk, 1997), citation impact factors, and the value of social work scholarship. A good place to start is publica-tion lag times. For example, of the 17 articles appearing in the April 2004 issue of *Social Work*, three were accepted for publication in 2000, five in 2001, eight in 2002, and only one in 2003. Therefore, most articles did not appear in print for 2-3 years following acceptance, while two articles ex-

126 *BIBLIOMETRICS IN SOCIAL WORK*

ceeded three years. If a reader wished to cite an article appearing in the April issue of *Social Work*, and submitted her manuscript to *Social Work* itself, it could easily take over two years before the article could be cited in print. This is important because a journal's 'impact factor' published by the Institute for Scientific Information is based on the numbers of times an article is cited *within two years of publication*. What this means, in effect, is that journals with longer publication lag times (those characteristic of many social work journals) have little chance of ever earning a high impact factor.

Another area of concern is the quality of peer review. As current or former editors of peer reviewed journals, we are fully aware of the potential to nurture many manuscripts to publication through helpful peer feedback. Far more attention needs to be paid to informing those who review manuscripts how to provide helpful feedback and the importance of doing so in a timely manner. See Epstein (in press) for one such study of how badly social work authors can be treated. A final area of concern is the plethora of journals that have evolved in our profession. Just as doubling the number of social work doctoral programs has not increased the numbers of doctoral level social workers, continuing to introduce new journal titles does not appear to improve the production, quality, or impact of scholarship in our profession. We would argue that fewer journals, with short review and publication cycles, offering quality peer review, with sustained circulation over time, would contribute to improving the quality of our scholarship.

It is difficult to say if bibliometrics makes a contribution to the social work profession, although it is hard to argue with the fact that as a profession our scholarship falls below other disciplines by various measures. The challenge is to improve by taking what we have learned and proceed now to implement measures to take the profession forward with respect to our research, publications, and other scholarly endeavors.

## REFERENCES

Dias, M. S. (1998). Publication patterns of the American society of pediatric neurosurgeons. *Pediatric Neurosurgery, 28*, 111-120.

Epstein, W. M. (in press). Confirmational response bias and the quality of the editorial processes among American social work journals. *Research on Social Work Practice*.

Gabbidon, S., & Green, H. T. (2001). The presence of African American scholarship in early American criminology texts (1918-1960). *Journal of Criminal Justice Education, 12*, 301-310.

Garfield, E. (1972). Citation analysis as a tool in journal evaluation. *Science, 178*, 471-479.

Green, R. G., Bellin, M. H., & Baskind, F. R. (2002). Results of the doctoral faculty publication project: Journal article productivity and its correlates in the 1990s. *Journal of Social Work Education, 38*, 135-152.

Griggs, R. A., & Proctor, D. L. (2002). A citation analysis of who's who in introductory textbooks. *Teaching of Psychology, 29*, 203-206.

Holden, G., Rosenberg, G., & Barker, K (2005a). Tracing thought through time and space: A selective review of bibliometrics in social work. *Social Work in Health Care, 41*(3/4), 1-34.

Holden, G., Rosenberg, G., & Barker, K (2005b). Bibliometrics: A potential decision making aid in hiring, reappointment, tenure and promotion decisions. *Social Work in Health Care, 41*(3/4), 67-92.

Koepke, J. M., & Thyer, B. A. (1985). Behavioral treatment of failure-to-thrive in a 2-year-old. *Child Welfare, 64*, 511-516.

Ligon, J., Thyer, B. A., & Dixon, D. (1995). Academic affiliations of those published in social work journals: A productivity analysis, 1989-1993. *Journal of Social Work Education, 31*, 369-376.

Perez, R. M., Constantine, M. G., & Gerard, P. (2000). Individual and institutional productivity of racial and ethnic minority research in the Journal of Counseling Psychology. *Journal of Counseling Psychology, 47*, 223-228.

Rosenberg, G., Holden, G., & Barker, K (2005). What happens to our ideas? A bibliometric analysis of articles in *Social Work in Health Care* in the 1990s. *Social Work in Health Care, 41*(3/4), 35-66.

Sims, J. L., & McGhee, N. J. (2003). Citation analysis and journal impact factors in ophthalmology and vision science journals. *Clinical and Experimental Ophthalmology, 31*, 12-22.

Stack, S. (2002). Gender and scholarly productivity: The case of criminal justice. *Journal of Criminal Justice, 30*, 175-182.

Sorensen, J. R. (1994). Scholarly productivity in criminal justice: Institutional affiliation of authors in the top ten criminal justice journals. *Journal of Criminal Justice, 22*, 535-547.

Taggart, W. A., & Holmes, M. D. (1991). Institutional productivity in criminal justice and criminology: An examination of author affiliation in selected journals. *Journal of Criminal Justice, 19*, 549-561.

Thyer, B. A. (1991). The enduring intellectual legacy of B. F. Skinner: A citation count from 1966-1989. *The Behavior Analyst, 14*, 73-75.

Thyer, B. A., Parrish, R. T., Curtis, G. C., Nesse, R. M., & Cameron, O. G. (1985). Ages of onset of DSM-III anxiety disorders. *Comprehensive Psychiatry, 16*, 111-115.

Thyer, B. A., & Polk, J. (1997). Social work and psychology professors' scholarly productivity: A controlled comparison of cited journal articles. *Journal of Applied Social Sciences, 21,* 105-110.

Wright, R. A. (2002). Recent changes in the most-cited scholars in criminal justice textbooks. *Journal of Criminal Justice, 30,* 183-105.

# Shallow Science or Meta-Cognitive Insights: A Few Thoughts on Reflection via Bibliometrics

Gary Holden, DSW
Gary Rosenberg, PhD
Kathleen Barker, PhD

**SUMMARY.** The authors conclude this volume by responding to the commentaries of their colleagues and reviewing relevant scholarship that appeared in the bibliometric literature since their literature reviews for the initial three articles in this issue were completed. They conclude, in part, that examination of bibliometric data regarding the entry of an article into the profession's knowledge base, and its ongoing life therein,

---

Gary Holden is Professor, New York University. Gary Rosenberg is Edith J. Baerwald Professor of Community and Preventive Medicine, Mount Sinai School of Medicine. Kathleen Barker is Professor of Psychology, The City University of New York: Medgar Evers College.

Address correspondence to: Gary Holden, DSW, Room 407, MC, 6112, New York University, School of Social Work, 1 Washington Square North, New York, NY 10003 (E-mail: gary.holden@nyu.edu).

[Haworth co-indexing entry note]: "Shallow Science or Meta-Cognitive Insights: A Few Thoughts on Reflection via Bibliometrics." Holden, Gary, Gary Rosenberg, and Kathleen Barker. Co-published simultaneously in *Social Work in Health Care* (The Haworth Social Work Practice Press, an imprint of The Haworth Press, Inc.) Vol. 41, No. 3/4, 2005, pp. 129-148; and: *Bibliometrics in Social Work* (ed: Gary Holden, Gary Rosenberg, and Kathleen Barker) The Haworth Social Work Practice Press, an imprint of The Haworth Press, Inc., 2005, pp. 129-148. Single or multiple copies of this article are available for a fee from The Haworth Document Delivery Service [1-800-HAWORTH, 9:00 a.m. - 5:00 p.m. (EST). E-mail address: docdelivery@haworthpress.com].

Available online at http://www.haworthpress.com/web/SWHC
© 2005 by The Haworth Press, Inc. All rights reserved.
doi:10.1300/J010v41n03_09

may provide insights about the scientific communication process that lead to improvements of that process. *[Article copies available for a fee from The Haworth Document Delivery Service: 1-800-HAWORTH. E-mail address: <docdelivery@haworthpress.com> Website: <http://www.HaworthPress.com> © 2005 by The Haworth Press, Inc. All rights reserved.]*

**KEYWORDS.** Bibliometrics, faculty, scholarship, informetrics, scientometrics, citation analysis, sociology of science, tenure, promotion

As preface to our reactions, we want to thank our colleagues for their insightful and reasoned commentaries on our work and the current state of affairs in bibliometrics. Individually and collectively, they have enhanced our undertaking on bibliometrics by raising issues and posing questions that we will respond to below. We will begin by addressing a general critique of the use of bibliometrics in social work. Then we will weave our responses to our colleagues comments into material that has either appeared since we wrote the three main articles in this volume or that we missed in our initial literature search. Our goal in doing this is to provide you with the most comprehensive and current view of bibliometrics in social work.

A broad criticism that has been raised regarding bibliometrics asks if it is simply 'keyboard driven, shallow science' (e.g., Kreuger, 1999). As Kreuger might inquire, are these bibliometric studies too remote from the basic mission of the profession? Perhaps. Bibliometric studies will not give us new incidence or prevalence data regarding new or existing conditions; nor will they describe the features of some new client population; nor will they tell us which practice intervention, research methodology or policy approach is most effective. Yet, are these the only questions a maturing field needs to ask?

As educators, it is important for us to understand what knowledge and which scholars appear to be having an impact on the larger community of scholars. Understanding the dissemination of knowledge and its acceptance by practitioners (translational research) has recently been a target of federal funding (e.g., Hudgins & Allen-Meares, 2000; National Institute of Mental Health, 2000). Understanding the dissemination and acceptance of knowledge by scholars is important as well. Why does some work enter into the discourse (as represented by citations) almost immediately, while other work reclines as virtual 'sleeping beauties' waiting to be discovered many years later (e.g., vanRaan, 2003)? Which scholars, journals, topics, and methodologies appear to have greater impact? Are there article structural factors, journal factors or author factors that predict impact (e.g., Meittunen & Nieminen, 2003)? Are there correctable biases in the publication process that can be discovered via bibliometric analyses? Are those in charge of the publication process (e.g., editorial boards) the most appropriate to carry out those responsibilities (e.g., Lindsey, 1976; 1992; Pardeck et al., 1991; Pardeck, 1992a; 1992b; 2002; Pardeck, Chung & Murphy, 1995; Pardeck & Meinart, 1999a; 1999b). What scholarship enters into the profession via the textbooks used by students (e.g., Christopher, Dobbins, Marek & Jones, 2004)? In general, bibliometric data regarding the entry of an article into the profession's knowledge base, and its ongoing life therein, may provide insights about the scientific communication process that lead to improvements of that process.

How can we improve the development and dissemination of knowledge without study? Take the data reported by Green (2005) in this issue. A question that arises is whether it is satisfactory for the profession to move ahead thinking all is well (or not well) with faculty scholarship? Social work faculty may have had the sense that we do not publish much–but nothing focuses our collective attention like an estimate of .28 articles per year. What explains this level of WoS article production? Although a multivariate explanation is obvious, it may be that social work faculty are writing and submitting articles for publication but that work is not being accepted for publication in WoS journals. If this assumption was true, faculty could, for instance, focus on improving the quality of the literature reviews conducted by doctoral graduates. This would likely lead to improved journal articles for years to come, and thus provide higher quality knowledge for practice. In our view, weak literature reviews in social work have been a self-limiting feature of the profession for years. Our hope is that by bringing additional data to the examination of social work scholarship via bibliometrics the field will improve its scholarship.

Although commenting on somewhat different facets of these topics, both Green (2005) and Ligon and Thyer (2005) ask if all of this effort on bibliometrics has real utility. One might ask in reponse: What would we know without the systematic information that bibliometrics has provided? Perhaps in the past a person who was relatively knowledgeable about social work scholarship might have known: that some journals, some authors, some schools, produced more articles than others; that some articles, some authors, some schools, were cited more frequently than others; that some editorial board members were publishing and being cited rather infrequently; etc. But there was probably no one in the field that knew all of the specifics and could convey them with the stark clarity that this accumulating body of bibliometrics data provides us. Is there utility beyond such clarity? While we know of no data related to the following we would assume that increased use of bibliometrics in social work has led, and will lead, to more effective library planning, more attention to publishing articles in journals of higher quality (as defined by ISI), and a concomitant decrease in publishing in non-peer reviewed venues, especially books done with proprietary publishers.[1]

## NEW AND PREVIOUSLY UNDISCOVERED BIBLIOMETRIC WORK

Since we finished writing the three primary articles in this special issue in January of 2004, the field of bibliometrics has moved forward. Although we had hoped to capture nearly all the work on bibliometrics in social work, we knew that we would not be able to cover all the potentially relevant articles in bibliometrics, and so therefore termed the review article a selective review (Holden, Rosenberg & Barker, 2005a). Since that time we have uncovered a few older articles that we missed and newer articles that have been published subsequently, which deserve mention.

New research has appeared that applies apply bibliometric analyses to a single journal (e.g., Quinones-Vidal, Lopez-Garcia, Penaranda-

Ortega & Tortosa-Gil, 2004), as we did in our examination of *Social Work in Health Care* (Rosenberg, Holden & Barker, 2005). Early in the review article, we included a brief overview of applications of bibliometrics to topics in social work beyond the productivity and impact of individuals and academic institutions. Subsequently, we also came across Thomas's (2000) study which demonstrates a local application of bibliometric techniques by a social work librarian. In an effort to provide empirical support for the library's journal acquisition decisions, Thomas examined masters degree theses at California State University: Long Beach (see Nicholson (2003) for a more general discussion of *bibliomining*). She found 22,183 references to 1,964 journals in her sample of theses. An important finding from a librarian's perspective was that almost 25% of the social work journals in the library were referenced less than ten times. The sad finding was that the 11th most frequently cited source was the Los Angeles Times.

In terms of the use of bibliometrics in studies of journals, Sellers, Mathiesen, Perry and Smith (2004) compared journal rankings across various indices: ISI impact factors scores (for the year 2000) and ratings of the quality and prestige (a combination of familiarity and quality rating used previously by Cnaan, Caputo & Shmuely, 1994). Utilizing a survey (n = 556, response rate = 26%) they examined 38 journals. Their data (extracted from Table 5) revealed statistically significant Spearman correlations of $r_s$ = .49 (p < .05) and .45 (p < .05) between the journals' impact factor score ranking and the rankings of journal quality and prestige, respectively. The authors state that "[t]his finding is not surprising because the two approaches differ in terms of focus, emphasis, and audience" (p. 156). They proceed to discuss the possible use of journal quality ratings by promotion and tenure committees. While we agree with Sellers, Mathiesen, Perry and Smith's spirit of multidimensional assessment for such decisions (and they do caution readers about using ratings as the main indicator of the quality of scholarship), we repeat Frank's (2003) admonition from earlier in this issue:

> Frank (2003) cautions us that because of inter- and intra-journal variations, citations to a scholar's articles are a better indicator of

that scholar's work than the impact factor of the journals in which they are published (c.f., Furr, 1995; Garfield, 1996; 1999; Seglen, 1997; Whitehouse, 2001). (Holden, Rosenberg & Barker, 2005b)

In general, using quality ratings of journals (especially when it is unclear as to what time period respondents are rating) based on low response rate surveys, done at specific points in time (compared to impact factor scores computed yearly) seems even more problematic than using impact factor scores as a proxy measure for the quality of a scholar's work. Using either group level measure (quality ratings of journals or impact factor scores) as a proxy measure of the quality of scholarship of an individual author risks an incorrect inference because of the *ecological fallacy* (i.e., inferring something about an individual based exclusively on data from a group to which they belong).

Puckett's (2003) report on a study of authors appeared after our search attempts were completed for the three primary articles in this issue. He examined publications and citations for the 1998-2000 period for 215 university based Australian social work authors and their schools. Puckett's group of most frequently cited authors ($n = 11$) received an average of 12.6 citations for the period (min.-max.: 5-41; literal self-citations were excluded). In terms of quantity of article productivity, this frequently cited group of authors published from 1 to 13 articles during the period.

Although we mentioned measurement problems in bibliometrics such as incorrect citation citations and spelling errors, we by no means fully explored this topic. Spivey and Wilks (2004) have opened a new line of inquiry in which they investigate the accuracy of reference lists in social work journals. They examined 100 references from five social work journals from the year 2000 (N = 500). They found that statistically significant differences in the number of errors per journal (*Social Service Review* had the lowest number of errors per reference). Conversely, they found no relationship between the age of the reference and errors, and no relationship between the number of authors (sole vs. multiple authorship) and errors. More recently, these authors have explored the perceptions of social work authors and editors regarding the accuracy of reference lists in journal articles (Wilks & Spivey, in press). This is clearly a line of research and possible intervention that would improve the validity of bibliometrics research.

## NEW RESEARCH ON PROBLEMATIC AREAS IN BIBLIOMETRICS

A number of the problematic areas in bibliometric research that we have noted in this issue have also received recent attention. We will now discuss a few of those in greater detail.

*Data sources.* In our review article we mentioned a number of the problematic issues associated with the data sources used in bibliometrics. Hood and Wilson (2003) have recently produced a more comprehensive and in depth treatment of these concerns. Although they tend to view the current state of the art as positive, they urge those doing bibliometric analyses to demand better data from the data sources they use (e.g., WoS, DIALOG). In fact, as we write this conclusion, we have begun to see announcements for a new database (Scopus from Elsevier) as well as changes to an existing data source (Thomson ISI's collaboration with NEC on a web citation index) that may mean substantial changes for bibliometric research (Hane, 2004; Quint, 2004). In a similar vein, Morrisey (2002) has made important suggestions regarding the development of *Uniform Author Identifiers* and *Uniform Concept Identifiers* that might improve the reliability and validity of bibliometric analyses.

*Scholarship coverage in the WoS.* While we pointed out potential sampling problems such as the fact that the WoS may not cover all the relevant journals or all of the volumes of journals that are included, we did not go as far in discussing these issues as Nisonger (2004). In this 'citation autobiography' Nisonger examined a variety of print and electronic sources as well as the web in order to determine the proportion of citations to his work in various venues. He reported that the WoS captured 44.6% of the citations appearing in print to his work (although as he notes this may be an overestimate because it may have not been possible to capture all citations outside of the WoS). Even though we don't know if this proportion would be similar to what we would find in social work, Nisonger's work serves as a reminder of this limitation of WoS based bibliometric analyses (c.f., Reid, 1995).

*Impact factor scores.* Journal impact factor scores are discussed in each of the three primary articles in this issue. They are defined and some of the pros and cons regarding their use are noted. Impact factor scores continue to prompt questions within bibliometrics though, and Garfield (2003) has recently published another set of responses to common questions about them. Although impact factors scores are determined in part by self-citations this topic has not been explored in social work to our knowledge (c.f., Anseel, Duyck & DeBaene, 2004–re: psychology).

*Self-citation.* In this issue, Klein and Bloom (2005) note concerns regarding self-citation. Although we have proposed an alternative definition of self citation when using bibliometrics to augment academic employment decisions (literal self-citation vs. co-author citation), the common view is employed by Glanzel, Thijs and Schlemmer (2004) in their recent work in this area–that is if the citing and the cited article share at least one author, it is considered a self-citation. Glanzel, Thijs and Schlemmer found, in part, that for 1999 WoS publications (using a three year citation window), that the bulk of the science publications had authors from the U.S. and the proportion of diachronous self-citations was lowest in the U.S. (22.1%). In a follow up study, examining WoS publications from 2000, Glanzel and Thijs (2004) found that the category of fields containing social work [Social Sciences I (General Regional & Community Issues)] had a diachronous self-citation rate of 23%.

Similarly, Gami, Montori, Wilczynski & Haynes (2004) examined citations to a sample of articles on diabetes published in the year 2000. The rates of diachronous self-citation were slightly less than those reported by Glanzel and Thijs for the U.S. for 1999 (mean 18%, median 7%; c.f., Kovacic & Misak, 2004).

The evidence from prior research including our own, combined with this new work strengthens our belief that the view noted by Glanzel, Thijs and Schlemmer (2004) is correct.

> In the bibliometric literature, there is an ongoing debate on the interpretation and role of author self-citations in the process of scientific communication. This debate has resulted in a certain polarisation. Particularly, users in science policy, but sometimes even the researchers themselves are condemning author self-citations as possible means of artificially inflating citation rates and thus of strengthening the authors' own positions in the scientific community. Bibliometricians are, on the other hand, inclined to regard a reasonable share of author self-citations as a natural part of scientific communication. According to this view, the almost absolute lack of self-citations over a longer period is just as pathological as an always-overwhelming share. (p. 63)

Based on their findings, Glanzel and Thijs (2004) conclude "at the macro level–there is no need for excluding self-citations in evaluative bibliometrics" (p. 310). We continue to believe that self-citations are often appropriate and therefore a less problematic aspect of bibliometrics than some authors assert. Regardless self citation is an aspect of scholarship that deserves further study in general as well as particular attention in academic employment decisions.

*Multiple authorship.* The issue of multiple authorship was addressed in our articles in this issue as it has been by many preceding authors. Trueba and Guerrero (2004) recently presented the development and testing of a new approach to this problem based on a view very similar to the view used in the development of our *Multiple Author Qualifier* (MAQ), which we apply to both authorship and citation counts. Their *Refined Weights* ($W_f$) approach differs from ours in the way they derive and test the credit assigned to authors at various positions, and also in that $W_f$ credits the first, second and last authors differently than the MAQ and more than their own "uncorrected" formulas would (these differences are clearest when there are more than four authors). Trueba

138                    BIBLIOMETRICS IN SOCIAL WORK

views this method as superior to the MAQ approach and also thinks that the calculation of the MAQ weights could be more precise (Personal Communication, 6/21/04).

While there has been some discussion about the possibility that senior authors may cede position to junior authors to help them out even though they were more substantial contributors than their authorship position conveys (c.f., Epstein, 2005), we have seen no evidence regarding this practice in social work. Furthermore, if it does occur, those senior authors should be discouraged from this practice because it violates an important norm of science that we discussed–that is that authorship credit should be assigned according to the relative contribution of the authors. To do otherwise simply clouds the reader's (and citation analysts') understanding.

*Theory.* While our articles spend virtually no space on theory of bibliometrics that does not mean that work is non-existent in this area. Beyond the references provided, the interested reader should see Small's (2004) recent tribute to Robert Merton, in which he continues Merton's normative view with his presentation of a citation classification system.[2]

*Meaning in bibliometrics.* In our review article we noted misspellings as well as factors such as authors who could "be citing work that is incorrect, not citing the best work, not correctly citing satisfactory work or may be failing to cite work that influenced them" that might present problems (Holden, Rosenberg & Barker, 2005a). As we were about to finish this manuscript a colleague gave us an intriguing paper to consider that suggests a problem we did not address directly (T. Festinger, Personal Communication, 5/4/04). Simkin and Roychowdhury (2003) report an application of bibliometrics as a challenge to bibliometrics (c.f., Simkin & Roychowdhury, 2004). Their reasoning is that if an incorrect citation is repeated in subsequent papers, those repeated mistakes represent instances where the citer did not read the original article. Morrisey (2002) has referred to these instances as *'hollow citations.'* Based on the analysis of a highly cited physics paper, Simkin and Roychowdhury conclude that: "[o]ur estimate is that only about 20% of citers read the original" (2003, p. 269). While we disagree with some of the premises and the conclusion of Simkin and Roychowdhury's work, they do a great service by raising yet another potential caution about the use of citation analysis. Even though they may not demonstrate the low level of reading primary documents that they claim, Simkin and Roychowdhury prompt us to reconsider what we think a citation indicates. How can we assume that a citation is an indicator of impact if the writer did not read the paper?

It goes back to the general question that a number of our colleagues in this issue raise in one form or another. What do these bibliometric measures mean (e.g., Epstein, 2005; Kirk, 2005; Klein & Bloom, 2005; Ligon & Thyer, 2005)? As with many constructs in the social sciences, we know that validity is an ongoing issue (c.f., Spriggs & Hansford (2000) for a discussion of the psychometric properties of Shepard's Citations for legal research). Aksnes and Taxt's (2004) recent findings regarding the positive relationship of bibliometric indicators to expert ratings builds on previous validity studies. Oppenheim's (1997) findings (which replicate his earlier studies) provide yet another example. He found high positive correlations between the U.K. Funding Council Research Assessment Exercise ratings (expert panel ratings where higher scores equal greater excellence) of university departments and the number of citations received. Regardless, more psychometric work on bibliometrics indicators is needed.

Klein and Bloom (2005) criticize our work on another measurement issue. They state:

> For example, these authors claim to assess "impact." And yet, even as they share that bibliometrics offers but one indicator, they are prompt in operationalizing this construct in terms of citations to a given work. The results of this operationalization may be an instance of what Donald Campbell has termed the "unmitigated disaster [of] the advice to employ designated operational definitions for theoretical terms" ... This process results in the richness of the term "impact" being reduced to an enumeration of citations. (p. 18)

We agree that operational definitions should be clearly distinguished from the concepts that spawned them. Operationalization involves moving from the concept to the specific indicators of the concept. On reflection, we think the problem described by Klein and Bloom is more the lack of clarity in our writing than in our operationalization of impact. In our review article (Holden, Rosenberg & Barker, 2005a), we stated that the focus is on *impact operationalized as citations to journal articles*. In that article we also state that "[c]itation analysis may not reflect the impact of unpublished scientific work or the impact a journal or article has on professionals who are reading it (but not writing and citing it)" (Table 1). Similarly, in that article we note:

> While the authors fully understand that impact can take many forms, in the current study it has been narrowly conceptualized as the impact of articles, operationalized as citations . . . That is, the number of articles that cite the target article. Criticisms of this approach will be considered in the Discussion section. . . . In terms of caveats, some readers may be thinking that the current study misses some of the impact produced by social workers' ideas. It does. Social workers' ideas have impact on the field via activities such as discussions with students and colleagues; teaching and supervision; presentations at a local, national or international conferences; publication in newsletters, monographs, books or in a variety of Internet outlets. But the mechanisms for studying the impact of such venues are less developed.

Impact does entail more than citations in the WoS–but any study circumscribes its focus. The article describing that study should explain the operationalization, the authors' justifications for the approach and the implications of those choices. Our work could have been more clearly explained.

It is clear that adding bibliometric analyses will not remove all subjectivity from academic employment decisions. But we do think that bibliometric analyses can help us to increase the ratio of empirical to subjective factors in these decisions. Kirk asks (2005):

... what is a personnel committee to make of the fact that a candidate's MAQ adjusted total cites per year is .77, or 1.77 or 2.77? Their usefulness is only in relation to some standard that may provide some meaning. We don't yet have such standards and so we are left with ambiguities. (p. 113)

Most approaches require a determination of the performance of an individual and dichotomous decision about that performance (e.g., hire/do not hire; tenure/do not tenure; promote/do not promote). There are always standards in the mind of the decision maker. Our complaint is that in the current situation there is excessive murkiness on both the performance assessment and the standards side. *Our proposal simply seeks to reduce the murkiness on the performance assessment side.* There are some normative data regarding faculty publications and citations in social work and more is needed (e.g., Bloom & Klein, 1995; Green, 1998; Green & Hayden, 2001; Green, Baskind & Bellin, 2002; Klein & Bloom, 1992; Rothman, Kirk & Knapp, 2003). Our suggestion is an incremental approach to the problem and we do recognize its limitations and set forth these limitations explicitly, for example, in the case of junior faculty (c.f., Klein & Bloom, 2005). Furthermore, we agree with Aksnes and Taxt:

Our results indicate that a bibliometric analysis can never function as a substitute for a peer review. However, a bibliometric analysis can counterbalance shortcomings and mistakes in peer judgments. In this way a bibliometric study should be considered as complementary to a peer evaluation. (p. 40)

*The future of bibliometrics in social work.* Along with methodological evolution comes topic evolution. Glanzel (2002) categorizes the current topical areas succinctly.

Present-day bibliometric research is aimed at the following three main target-groups that clearly determine topics and sub-areas of "contemporary bibliometrics."

142 *BIBLIOMETRICS IN SOCIAL WORK*

*Bibliometrics for Bibliometricians ("Basic Research" in Bibliometrics)*

This is the domain of basic bibliometric research and is traditionally funded by the usual grants. Methodological research is conducted mainly in this domain.

*Bibliometrics for Scientific Disciplines (Scientific Information)*

The researchers in scientific disciplines form the bigger, but also the most diverse interest-group in bibliometrics. Due to their primary scientific orientation, their interests are strongly related to their specialty. . . .

*Bibliometrics for Science Policy and Management (Research Evaluation)*

This is the domain of *research evaluation*, at present the most important topic in the field. Here the national, regional, and institutional structures of science and their comparative presentation are in the foreground. (no p.)

Increased use of bibliometrics will likely bring a number of outcomes, including:

1. evolution of bibliometric methods (c.f., Klein & Bloom, 2005);
2. increased sophistication of critiques; and
3. changed citation behavior in the scholarly literature.

Consider this third potential outcome. Science moves forward aided by the corrective influence of professional norms including personal, professional society and funding agency sanctions for misconduct (c.f., Merton, 2000). As new or old methods (e.g., bibliometrics) are employed, certain types of misconduct may be illuminated. While we have suggested increased use of bibliometrics for hiring, retention, promotion and tenure decisions (Holden, Rosenberg & Barker, 2005b), we are well aware that such calls may prompt misconduct, as some individuals might try to influence the outcome of such decisions by engaging in inappropriate citation behavior. Yet at the same time, more refined bibliometric methods will provide more precise descriptions of authors' citation behavior. While the motivation to cheat the system may increase as use of our system (or other systems) increases, increased use and refinement of such systems would similarly increase the chances of detecting cheaters and thereby reduce motivating for cheating. For instance, in this volume we introduced both a refined citation statistic (self-citation split into literal self-citation and co-author citation), as well as the MAQ adjustment for multiple authorship in response to issues like 'inappropriate self-citation' and 'inappropriate assignment of authorship.' For instance, if committees routinely used the MAQ, authors would have less motivation to get themselves added as additional authors on multi-authored articles. While having some superficial logic it remains to be seen if this discussion represents anything more than idle speculation.

Kirk (2005) and Green (2005) ask the important question that all of our colleagues ask directly or indirectly. That is, will the proposed method that is designed to improve academic employment decisions actually do so? As comments within this volume demonstrates, tenure criteria linked to bibliometrics elicits a range of reactions but caution appears to be commonly threaded throughout. At the same time, it is notable that there is an unhappiness expressed in terms publishing and social work's scholarly productivity. These concerns are hardly accidental and demonstrate an underlying tension in the evaluation of productivity. In our view, productivity in academe should not be measured strictly by "counting," or with other measures that are similarly corporate in nature. Academe exists so that smart people can "think" about the world, reflect, and write. We believe that bibliometric methods are a natural extension of those activities. Still, more research is needed to better understand the actual utility of these methods.

In conclusion, while continued growth and development of bibliometric research outside of the field of social work seems probable, the likelihood of such growth within the field is uncertain. We hope that our efforts and the thoughtful comments of our colleagues in this volume will add to the knowledge base that social work researchers will use to make decisions about whether or not to pursue bibliometric studies in the future. We look forward to learning what happens to these ideas.

## NOTES

1. This last possibility is perhaps the most important, because until academics focus their publication efforts on peer reviewed articles in venues which can be wrested from the grip of the for profit-publishers (see Harnad (2001) re: university based pre-print servers), we will continue to have less control over the scholarly publication process than we rightly deserve given that we are discussing *our intellectual product*.

2. We found Epstein's (2005) comments about Merton consonant with others' allegories. Although exploration of Merton's conceptual contributions to bibliometrics is beyond the scope of this article, it should be noted here that Cole (2004) has just reported data that demonstrates that Merton was larger than life.

A few years later when I was his teaching assistant, it occurred to me and to his other students that Merton seemed larger than life. Consistent with my training, I tested that hypothesis in a survey of students in that course, Analysis of Social Structures. Over 150 responded to the question: How tall is Robert K. Merton? There was little variance in opinion. The class average had Merton at 6 feet 3 and a-half inches in height–a full two inches taller than he actually was. It was true. Merton was, in fact, larger than life. (Cole, 2004, p. 39)

## REFERENCES

Aksnes, D. W. & Taxt, R. E. (2004). Peer reviews and bibliometric indicators: A comparative study at a Norwegian university. *Research Evaluation, 13, 1,* 33-41.

Anseel, F., Duyck, W. & DeBaene, W. (2004). Journal impact factors and self-citations: Implications for psychology journals. *American Psychologist, 59, 1,* 49-51.

Bloom, M. & Klein, W. C. (1995). Publications & citations: A study of faculty at leading schools of social work. *Journal of Social Work Education, 31,* 377-387.

Christopher, A. N., Dobbins, E. M., Marek, P. & Jones, J. R. (2004). Three decades of social psychology: A longitudinal analysis of Baron and Byrne's textbook. *Teaching of Psychology, 31, 1,* 31-36.

Cnaan, R. A., Caputo, R. K. & Shmuely, Y. (1994). Senior faculty perceptions of social work journals. *Journal of Social Work Education, 30,* 185-199.

Cole, J. R. (2004). Robert K. Merton, 1910-2003. *Scientometrics, 60, 1,* 37-40.

Epstein, I. (2005). Following in the footnotes of giants: Citation analysis and its discontents. *Social Work in Health Care, 41*(3/4), 93-101.

Fischer, J. (1973). Is casework effective–review. *Social Work, 18.*

Gami, A. S., Montori, V. M., Wilczynski, N. L. & Haynes, R. B. (2004). Author self-citation in the diabetes literature. *Canadian Medical Association Journal, 170, 13.* Retrieved 6/25/04 from: http://www.cmaj.ca/cgi/content/full/170/13/1925

Garfield, E. (2003). The meaning of the Impact Factor. *International Journal of Clinical and Health Psychology, 3, 2,* 363-369.

Glanzel, W. (2002). A concise introduction to bibliometrics & its history. Retrieved 5/15/04 from: http://www.steunpuntoos.be/bibliometrics.html

Glanzel, W. & Thijs, B. (2004). The influence of author self-citations on bibliometric macro indicators. *Scientometrics, 59, 3,* 281-310.

Glanzel, W., Thijs, B. & Schlemmer, B. (2004). A bibliometric approach to the role of author self-citations in scientific communication. *Scientometrics, 59, 1,* 63-77.

Green, R. G. (1998). Faculty rank, effort, and success: A study of publication in professional journals. *Journal of Social Work Education, 34,* 415-427.

Green, R. G. & Hayden, M. A. (2001). Citation of articles published by the most productive social work faculties in the 1990's. *Journal of Social Service Research, 27, 3,* 41-56.

Green, R. G., Baskind, F. R. & Bellin, M. H. (2002). Results of the doctoral faculty publication project: Journal article productivity and its correlates in the 1990s. *Journal of Social Work Education, 37,* 135-152.

Green, R. G. (2005). The paradox of faculty publications in professional journals. *Social Work in Health Care,* 41(3/4).

Hane, P. J. (2004). Elsevier announces Scopus service. Retrieved 5/12/04 from: http://infotoday.mondosearch.com/cgi-bin/MsmGo.exe?grab_id=20&EXTRA_A RG=&CFGNAME=MssFind%2Ecfg&host_id=42&page_id=1770752&query=sc opus&hiword=scopus+#top

Harnad, S. (2001). For whom the gate tolls? How and why to free the refereed research literature online through author/institution self-archiving, now. Retrieved 6/1/04 from: http://www.cogsci.soton.ac.uk/~harnad/Tp/resolution.htm

Holden, G., Rosenberg, G. & Barker, K (2005a). Tracing thought through time and space: A selective review of bibliometrics in social work. *Social Work in Health Care,* 41(3/4), 1-34.

Holden, G., Rosenberg, G. & Barker, K (2005b). Bibliometrics: A potential decision making aid in hiring, reappointment, tenure and promotion decisions. *Social Work in Health Care,* 41(3/4), 67-92.

Hood, W. W. & Wilson, C. S. (2003). Informetric studies using databases: Opportunities and challenges. *Scientometrics, 58, 3,* 587-608.

Hudgins, C. A. & Allen-Meares, P. (2000). Translational research: A new solution to an old problem. *Journal of Social Work Education, 36,* 103-114.

Kirk, S. (2005). Politics of personnel and landscapes of knowledge. *Social Work in Health Care,* 41(3/4), 109-116.

Klein, W. C. & Bloom, M. (1992). Studies of scholarly productivity in social work using citation analysis. *Journal of Social Work Education, 28,* 291-299.

146 BIBLIOMETRICS IN SOCIAL WORK

Klein & Bloom (2005). Bibliometrics: The best available information? *Social Work in Health Care, 41*(3/4) 117-121.

Kovacic, N. & Misak, A. (2004). Author self-citation in medical literature. *Canadian Medical Association Journal, 170*, 13. Retrieved 6/25/04 from: http://www.cmaj.ca/cgi/content/full/170/13/1929

Kreuger, L. W. (1999). Shallow science? *Research on Social Work Practice, 9*, 108-110.

Ligon, J. & Thyer, B. A. (2005). Bibliometrics and social work: A two-edged sword can still be a blunt instrument. *Social Work in Health Care, 41*(3/4), 123-128.

Lindsey, D. (1976). Distinction, achievement and editorial board membership. *American Psychologist, 31*, 799-804.

Lindsey, D. (1978). *The scientific publication system in social science.* San Francisco: Jossey-Bass.

Lindsey, D. (1992). Improving the quality of social work journals: From the Editor of *Children and Youth Services Review. Research on Social Work Practice, 2*, 515-524.

Meittunen, J. & Nieminen, P. (2003). The effect of statistical methods and study reporting characteristics on the number of citations: A study of four general psychiatric journals. *Scientometrics, 57*, 377-88.

Merton, R. K. (2000). On the Garfield input to the sociology of science: A retrospective collage. In B. Cronin & H. B. Atkins (Eds.), *The Web of Knowledge: A Festschrift in Honor of Eugene Garfield* (pp. 435-448). Medford, NY: Information Today.

Morrisey, L. J. (2002). Bibliometric and bibliographic analysis in an era of electronic scholarly communication. *Science & Technology Libraries, 22, 3/4*, 149-160.

National Institute of Mental Health (2000). Translating behavioral science into action. Retrieved 5/14/04, from: http://www.nimh.nih.gov/publicat/nimhtranslating.pdf

Nicholson, S. (2003). The bibliomining process: Data warehousing and data mining for library decision making. *Information Technology and Libraries, 22, 4*, 146-151.

Nisonger, T.E. (2004). Citation autobiography: An investigation of ISI database coverage in determining author citedness. *College & Research Libraries* v. 65 no. 2 152-163.

Oppenheim, C. (1997). The correlation between citation counts and the 1992 research assessment exercise ratings for British research in genetics, anatomy and archaeology. *Journal of Documentation, 53*, 477-487.

Pardeck, J. T., Arndt, B. J., Light, D. B., Mosley, G. F., Thomas, S. D., Werner, M. A. & Wilson, K. E. (1991). Distinction and achievement levels of editorial board members of psychology and social work journals. *Psychological Reports, 68*, 523-27.

Pardeck, J. T. (1992a). Are social work journal editorial boards competent? Some disquieting data with implications for research on social work practice. *Research on Social Work Practice, 2*, 487-96.

Pardeck, J. T. (1992b). The distinction and achievement levels of social work editorial boards revisited. *Research on Social Work Practice, 2*, 529-537.

Pardeck, J. T. (2002). Scholarly productivity of editors of social work and psychology journals. *Psychological Reports*, *90*, 1051-1054.

Pardeck, J. T., Chung, W. S. & Murphy, J. W. (1995). An examination of the scholarly productivity of social work journal editorial board members and guest reviewers. *Research on Social Work Practice*, *5*, 223-234.

Pardeck, J. T. & Meinart, R. G. (1999a). Scholarly achievements of the *Social Work* editorial board and consulting editors: A commentary. *Research on Social Work Practice*, *9*, 86-91.

Pardeck, J. T. & Meinart, R. G. (1999b). Improving the scholarly quality of *Social Work's* editorial board and consulting editors: A professional obligation. *Research on Social Work Practice*, *9*, 121-127.

Quinones-Vidal, E., Lopez-Garcia, J. J., Penaranda-Ortega, M. & Tortosa-Gil, F. (2004). The nature of social and personality psychology as reflected in JPSP, 1965-2000. *Journal of Personality and Social Psychology*, *83*, *3*, 435-152.

Quint, B. (2004). Thomson ISI to track web-based scholarship with NEC's CiteSeer. Retrieved 5/12/04 from: http://www.infotoday.com/newsbreaks/nb 040301-1.shtml

Reid, K. L. (1995). Citation analysis of faculty publication: Beyond *Science Citation Index and Social Science Citation Index*. *Bulletin of the Medical Library Association*, *83*, *4*, 503-508.

Rosenberg, G., Holden, G. & Barker, K (2005). What happens to our ideas? A bibliometric analysis of articles in *Social Work in Health Care* in the 1990s. *Social Work in Health Care*, *41*(3/4), 35-66.

Rothman, J., Kirk, S. A. & Knapp, H. (2003). Reputation and publication productivity among social work researchers. *Social Work Research*, *27*, 105-115.

Sellers, S. L., Mathiesen, S. G., Perry, R. & Smith, T. (2004). Evaluation of social work journal quality: Citation versus reputation approaches. *Journal of Social Work Education*, *40*, *1*, 143-160.

Simkin, M. V. & Roychodhury, V. P. (2003). Read before you cite! *Complex Systems*, *14*, 269-74.

Simkin, M. V. & Roychodhury, V. P. (2004). Stochastic modeling of citation slips. Retrieved 5/6/04 from: *http://arxiv.org/abs/cond-mat/0401529*

Small, H. (2004). On the shoulders of Robert Merton: Towards a normative theory of citation. *Scientometrics*, *60*, *1*, 71-79.

Spriggs, J. F. & Hansford, T. G. (2000). Measuring legal change: The reliability and validity of *Shepard's Citations*. *Political Research Quarterly*, *53*, *2*, 327-41.

Spivey, C. A. & Wilks, S. E. (2004). Reference list accuracy in social work journals. *Research on Social Work Practice*, *14*, *4*, 281-286.

*148*  *BIBLIOMETRICS IN SOCIAL WORK*

Thomas, J. (2000). Never enough: Graduate student use of journals–citation analysis of social work theses. *Behavioral and Social Sciences Librarian, 19, 1,* 1-16.

Trueba, F. J. & Guerrero, H. (2004). A robust formula to credit authors for their publications. *Scientometrics, 60, 2,* 181-204.

vanRaan, A. F. J. (2003). Sleeping beauties in science. *Scientometrics, 59, 3,* 467-472.

Wilks, S. E. & Spivey, C. A., (in press). Views of reference list accuracy from social work journal editors and published authors.

# Index

Page numbers followed by the letter "t" designate tables. *See also* cross-references designate related topics.

Academic freedom, 85-86
Academics, quality of venue and, 57
Academic *vs.* practice fields, 22
Accuracy, of reference lists, 134-135
Adjusted total articles, 84
Advantages and disadvantages, 4,5-6t
Age of articles, 41
    computation of, 76-77
    *Social Work in Health Care*, 50,
        51-54t,55
American Society of Pediatric
        Neurosurgeons, 124
Applications
    of citation analysis, 3,7-8,114
    library, 133
Appropriate *vs.* inappropriate
        self-citation, 42
Associate/assistant professors,
        frequency of citation, 71
Audit culture, 85
Authors
    Australian, 134
    impact of, 24
    number of, 43,44t,56,78-79. *See*
        *also* Multiple authorship

Best available information principle,
        117-121
Bias, 6t
    in self-citation, 6t
Bibliometrics. *See also* Citation
        analysis
    advantages, 4,5-6t
    applications, 3,114

basic research, 142
in decision-making, 67-102
definitions, 70-72
disadvantages, 4,4t
future in social work, 141-144
journals related to, 3
lack of standards, 113-114,141
library applications, 133
meaning, 119,138-139. *See also*
    Critiques
new research, 135-144
personal memoir (I. Epstein),
    93-101
research evaluation, 142
scientific information, 142
shortcomings, 79-86,117-121. *See*
    *also* Critiques
single-journal analyses, 132-133
in social work specifically, 7-8
theoretical base, 2-3
utility of, 132. *See also* Critiques
Bibliomining, 133
Bloom, Martin, critique of current
    study, 117-121
*British Journal of Social Work*, impact,
    24,39

(University of) Califormia–Los
        Angeles, critique of current
        study (S. Kirk), 119-121
(University of) California–Berkeley, 25
Circulation, 38,81-82
Citation analysis
    definitions, 3,69

150                 BIBLIOMETRICS IN SOCIAL WORK

meaning, 119,138-139. *See also*
     Critiques
Citation context, 80
Citation indexing, 3-4
Citations
     hollow, 138-139
     incorrect, 80-81,134-135,138-139
     number of, 50,71
     pattern variations, 81
Citedness, 42,79
City University of New York: Medgar
     Evers College, 1-31,35-66,
     67-102,129-148
Columbia University, 25
Concentration, 42
(University of) Connecticut, critique of
     current study (Klein &
     Bloom), 117-121
Content analysis, 80
Context, citation, 80
Contribution *vs.* quality, 19
Core influence, 60
Corrected quality ratios, 19,76
Council on Social Work Education,
     credit assignment
     recommendations, 84
Counts
     adjusted, 84
     adjusted total articles, 84
     normal (whole), 83-84,85
Coverage limitations, 81
Credit assignment, 83-84. *See also*
     Multiple authorship
     normal (whole) counts, 85
     in psychology, 84
Criminal justice studies, 124
Criticisms
     academic freedom issues, 85-86
     audit culture concept, 85-86
     relevance of, 79-80
Critiques
     Florida State University (Ligon, J.),
          123-128
     Georgia State University (B.
          Thyer), 123-128

responses to, 129-148
University of California–Los
     Angeles (S. Kirk), 109-121
University of Connecticut (Klein &
     Bloom), 117-121
Virginia Commonwealth University
     (R. Green), 103-108


Data analysis, 20
Databases
     *Arts & Humanities Citation Index,*
          72
     Price Index, 77
     *Science Citation Expanded,* 72
     Scopus database (Elsevier), 135
     Shepard's Citations, 139
     *Social Science Citation Index*
          (SSCI), 8,9-17t
     Thomson ISI/NEC collaboration,
          135
     Web of Science (WoS), 18,38,58,
          135-136
Data sources, new research, 135
Decision-making, 67-102
     approach to study, 72,73-75t
     conclusion, 86
     problems with bibliometrics, 79-86
Definitions, operational, 18-19
Diabetes articles, self-citation, 136
Diachronous self-citation, 42,59,
     77-78,82-83
Distribution, skewed. *See* Skewed
     distribution
Drug and alcohol journals, impact, 39
Duration of study, 57-58


Ecological fallacy, 134
Editors, impact of, 20-23
*Encyclopedia of Social Work,* 24,71
Epstein, J., personal memoir, 93-101
Errors per journal, 134-135

*Index*

151

Faculty, impact of, 24-26
Florida State University, critique of
    current study (Ligon, J.),
    123-128
Freud, Sigmund, citations, 124
Full professors, frequency of citation, 71
Funding, for translational research, 130

Generalizability, 58-59
Georgia State University, critique of
    current study (B. Thyer),
    123-128
Green, Robert G., critique of currrent
    study, 103-108

High impact groups, *Social Work in
    Health Care*, 44,45-49t
Hollow citations, 138-139
Hunter College of Social Work, 93-101

Ideas, 57
    *vs.* citations, 115-116
Impact, 19-26
    of authors, 24
    *British Journal of Social Work,* 39
    core influence, 60
    critique of definition, 119
    critiques of, 139-140
    defining, 125
    drug and alcohol journals, 39
    duration of study and, 57-58
    of editors, 20-23
    of faculty, 24-26
    of journal articles, 39-40
    of journals, 23,37-38
    new studies, 133-134
    number of authors and, 56
    number of pages and, 56
    number of references and, 56
    of readers *vs.* citers, 59

*Social Work in Health Care*, 35-66,
    44,45-49t. *See also Social
    Work in Health Care*
    statistical method and, 56-57
    study design and, 56
    *vs.* quality, 19
Impact factor score, 23,38,82,133
    new research, 136
Incorrect citations, 134-135,138-139
Incorrect referencing, 58,80-81
Incorrect work, 58,80-81
Indexing, citation, 3-4
Indicators, psychometric properties, 23
Informal influences, 6t
Informetrics, 2
Institute for Scientific Information
    (ISI), 38
    recommendations of, 7
Inter-discipline comparisons, 124-125
    *Social Work in Health Care*, 55-56
    social-work *vs.* non-social work
    articles, 72
Inter-institutional comparisons, 4
Interpretation, ISI recommendations, 7
Interprofessional contrasts, 25

Journal articles, impact, 39-40
Journals
    bibliometrics-related, 3
    circulation, 81-82
    coverage limitations, 81
    errors per journal, 134-135
    impact of, 23,37-38
    new studies, 133-134
    numbers studied, 80
    specialized, 81-82
    technical limitations, 81
    as unit of analysis, 38

Kendal's tau, 43
Kirk, Stuart A., critique of current
    study, 109-121

Klein, Waldo C., critique of current study, 117-121

Lag time, 41,77,80,125-126
Length of article, 43,44t
Library applications, 133
Ligon, Jan, critique of current study, 123-128
Lotka's Law of Scientific Productivity of Authors, 18

Meaning, 119,138-139. *See also* Critiques
Mean number of references, 55
Metrics
problems with, 134-135
types of, 2
Mount Sinai School of Medicine, 1-31, 35-66,67-102,129-148
Multiple Author Qualifier (MAQ), 76, 78t,85,113-114,143
new research, 137-138
Multiple authorship, 6t
credit assignment, 83-84
new research, 137-138
*Social Work in Health Care*, 43-44, 55

New research, 132-144
data sources, 135
impact factor scores, 136
on meaning, 138-139
multiple authorship, 137-138
scholarship on WoS, 135-136
self-citation, 136-137
theory, 138
New York University, 1-31,35-66, 67-102,129-148
Normal (whole) counts, 83-84,85
Number
of articles, 43,44t

of authors, 43,44t,56,78-79. *See also* Multiple authorship
of citations, 50
full *vs.* associate/assistant professors, 71
social-work *vs.* non-social work articles, 72
of journals studied, 80
of pages, 56

Operational definitions, 18-19
Operationalization, 118,139-140

Pages, number of, 56
Peer review, 23,126,141,144
Persistence, 77
Personal memoir (I. Epstein), 93-101
Pertinence, 41
Physicists' publications, 19
Piaget, Jean, citations, 124
Practice *vs.* academic fields, 22
Practitioners *vs.* researchers, scholarship of, 26
Prestige, 133
Principal authorship. *See* Credit assignment; Multiple authorship
Productivity, 8,9-17t,19
*Social Work* editorial board, 21-22
Psychology
credit assignment rules, 84
editorial board productivity, 22
introductory text study, 124-125
*vs.* social work, 20
Psychometric properties, of indicators, 23

Quality, 6t
corrected quality ratios, 19,76
defining, 125
of literature reviews, 131

# Index

new research, 133-134
of venue, 57
*vs.* contribution, 19
*vs.* impact, 19

Quantity, 8,9-17t,19

Ranking, 71
References
  accuracy of lists, 134-135
  mean number of, 55
  *Social Work in Health Care*, 55
Refined Weights, 137
Relevance, 5t
Researchers *vs.* practitioners,
    scholarship of, 26
*Research on Social Work Practice*, 20

Sampling, 5t,18-19
Scholarship, practitioners *vs.*
    researchers, 26
*Science Citation Expanded*, 72
Scopus database (Elsevier), 135
Self-citation, 6t,21,59
  appropriate *vs.* inappropriate, 42
  diabetes articles, 136
  diachronous, 42,59,77-78,82-83
  evaluation of, 82-83
  new research, 136-137
  *Social Work in Health Care,* 42
  synchronous, 42,82,83
Self-reports, 58
Shepard's Citations, psychometric
    properties, 139
Situation analysis, 3-4
Skewed distributions, 6t,20,80
Skinner, B.F., citations, 124
*Social Science Citation Index* (SSCI),
    8,9-17t
*Social Science Review*

circulation, 81-82
errors per reference, 134
*Social Sciences Citation Index*, 72
Social work
  disadvantages related to, 6t
  editorial board productivity, 22
  low publication rate, 131
  *vs.* psychology, 20
*Social Work*
  circulation, 81-82
  editorial board productivity, 21-22
  impact, 24
  impact factor score, 23,38
  lag time, 125-126
*Social Work in Health Care*, 35-66
  age of articles, 50,51-54t,55
  background of study, 36-37
  discussion, 55-60
  high impact groups, 44,45-49t
  impact, 44,45-49t
  impact factor score, 38
  impact of journals generally, 37-38
  inter-field comparisons, 55-56
  length of article, 43,44t
  mean number of references, 55
  measures, 41-42
  method, 40-42
  multiple authorship, 55
  number of authors, 43,44t
  number of citations, 50
  number of references, 43,44t
  procedure, 41
  results, 42-55,44t,45-49t,51-54t
  sample, 40,42-43
  time frame, 40
Specialized journals, 81-82
Spelling errors, 134
Standards, lack of, 113-114,141
Study design, 56,72,73-75t
  relevance of, 58
Subjectivity, 69,71,109-121
Submission–publication time. *See* Lag
    times
Synchronous self-citation, 42,82,83

Technical limitations, 5t,81
Tenure, quality of venue and, 57
Theoretical base, 2-3
Theory, new research, 138
Thyer, Bruce A., critique of current
  study, 123-128
Translational research, 130-131
Trends, 6t


U.K. Funding Council Research
  Assessment Exercise, 139
*Uniform Author Identifiers and
  Uniform Concept Identifiers*
  (Morrisey), 135
Units of analysis, journals as, 38
University of California–Berkeley, 25
University of California–Los Angeles,
  critique of current study (S.
  Kirk), 109-121
University of Connecticut, critique of
  current study (Klein &
  Bloom), 117-121
University of Washington–Seattle, 25

University of Wisconsin, 25
Unpublished work, omission of, 6t


Venue, quality of, 57
Virginia Commonwealth University,
  critique of current study,
  103-108
Virginia University *Doctored Faculty
  Decade Publication Project*,
  68


(University of) Washington–Seattle, 25
Washington University, 25
Web, citation analysis and, 3-4
Web of Science (WoS), 18,38
  new research, 135-136
  number of journals, 58
Whole (normal) counts, 83-84,85
(University of) Wisconsin, 25

# BOOK ORDER FORM!

Order a copy of this book with this form or online at:
http://www.HaworthPress.com/store/product.asp?sku= 5711

## Bibliometrics in Social Work

____ in softbound at $17.95 ISBN-13: 978-0-7890-3071-9 / ISBN-10: 0-7890-3071-3.
____ in hardbound at $24.95 ISBN-13: 978-0-7890-3070-2 / ISBN-10: 0-7890-3070-5.

COST OF BOOKS ____

POSTAGE & HANDLING ____
US: $4.00 for first book & $1.50
for each additional book
Outside US: $5.00 for first book
& $2.00 for each additional book.

SUBTOTAL ____
In Canada: add 7% GST. ____

STATE TAX ____
CA, IL, IN, MN, NJ, NY, OH, PA & SD residents
please add appropriate local sales tax.

FINAL TOTAL ____
If paying in Canadian funds, convert
using the current exchange rate,
UNESCO coupons welcome.

❏ BILL ME LATER:
Bill-me option is good on US/Canada/
Mexico orders only; not good to jobbers,
wholesalers, or subscription agencies.

❏ Signature ____

Payment Enclosed: $ ____

❏ PLEASE CHARGE TO MY CREDIT CARD:
❏ Visa ❏ MasterCard ❏ AmEx ❏ Discover
❏ Diner's Club ❏ Eurocard ❏ JCB

Account # ____

Exp Date ____

Signature ____
(Prices in US dollars and subject to change without notice.)

PLEASE PRINT ALL INFORMATION OR ATTACH YOUR BUSINESS CARD

Name

Address

City          State/Province          Zip/Postal Code

Country

Tel          Fax

May we use your e-mail address for confirmations and other types of information? ❏ Yes ❏ No We appreciate receiving your e-mail address. Haworth would like to e-mail special discount offers to you, as a preferred customer.
**We will never share, rent, or exchange your e-mail address.** We regard such actions as an invasion of your privacy.

Order from your **local bookstore** or directly from
**The Haworth Press, Inc.** 10 Alice Street, Binghamton, New York 13904-1580 • USA
Call our toll-free number (1-800-429-6784) / Outside US/Canada: (607) 722-5857
Fax: 1-800-895-0582 / Outside US/Canada: (607) 771-0012
E-mail your order to us: orders@HaworthPress.com

**For orders outside US and Canada,** you may wish to order through your local
sales representative, distributor, or bookseller.
For information, see http://HaworthPress.com/distributors

(Discounts are available for individual orders in US and Canada only, not booksellers/distributors.)

**Please photocopy this form for your personal use.**
www.HaworthPress.com

BOF06